Surviving Identity

CW00521496

Today, political claims are increasingly made on the basis of experienced trauma and inherent vulnerability, as evidenced in the growing number of people who identify as a 'survivor' of one thing or another, and also in the way in which much political discourse and social policy assumes the vulnerability of the population. This book discusses these developments in relation to the changing focus of social movements, from concerns with economic redistribution towards campaigns for cultural recognition. As a result of this, the experience of trauma and psychological vulnerability has become a dominant paradigm within which both personal and political grievances are expressed.

Combining the psychological, social and political aspects of the expression of individual distress and political dissent, this book provides a unique analysis of how concepts such as 'vulnerability' and 'trauma' have become institutionalized within politics and society, and also offers a critical appraisal of the political and personal implications of these developments. In addition, the book shows how the institutionalization of the survivor identity represents a diminished view of the human subject and our capacity to achieve progressive political and individual change.

This book will be of interest to researchers, postgraduates and undergraduate students of critical psychology, sociology, social policy, politics, social movements and mental health.

Kenneth McLaughlin is a senior lecturer in social work at Manchester Metropolitan University. He has extensive experience in social work and social care as a support worker for homeless families and as a social worker in a local authority statutory mental health team.

Concepts for Critical Psychology: Disciplinary Boundaries Re-thought
Series editor: Ian Parker

Developments inside psychology that question the history of the discipline and the way it functions in society have led many psychologists to look outside the discipline for new ideas. This series draws on cutting edge critiques from just outside psychology in order to complement and question critical arguments emerging inside. The authors provide new perspectives on subjectivity from disciplinary debates and cultural phenomena adjacent to traditional studies of the individual.

The books in the series are useful for advanced level undergraduate and postgraduate students, researchers and lecturers in psychology and other related disciplines such as cultural studies, geography, literary theory, philosophy, psychotherapy, social work and sociology.

Forthcoming Titles:

Drugs, Gender and the Social Imaginary
By Ilana Mountian

Psychologisation in Times of Globalisation
By Jan De Vos

Self Research
The Intersection of Therapy and Research
By Ian Law

Surviving Identity

Vulnerability and the Psychology of Recognition

Kenneth McLaughlin

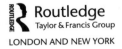
Routledge
Taylor & Francis Group

LONDON AND NEW YORK

First published 2012
by Routledge
27 Church Road, Hove, East Sussex BN3 2FA

Simultaneously published in the USA and Canada
by Routledge
711 Third Avenue, New York NY 10017

*Routledge is an imprint of the Taylor & Francis Group, an informa
business*

© 2012 Psychology Press

British Library Cataloguing in Publication Data
A catalogue record for this book is available from the British Library

Library of Congress Cataloging-in-Publication Data
McLaughlin, Kenneth.
  Surviving identity : vulnerability and the psychology of recognition /
Kenneth McLaughlin. – 1st ed.
      p. cm. – (Concepts for critical psychology: disciplinary
boundaries re-thought)
  Includes bibliographical references and index.
  ISBN 978-0-415-59120-1 (hardback) – ISBN 978-0-415-59121-8
(pbk.) 1. Social movements–Psychological aspects. 2. Action research.
3. Psychic trauma. 4. Identity (Psychology) I. Title.
  HM881.M435 2012
  303.48'401–dc23

                                                    2011024530

ISBN: 978-0-415-59120-1 (hbk)
ISBN: 978-0-415-59121-8 (pbk)
ISBN: 978-0-203-14766-5 (ebk)

Typeset in Times by Garfield Morgan, Swansea, West Glamorgan
Paperback cover design by Andrew Ward
Printed and bound in Great Britain by TJ International Ltd, Padstow,
Cornwall

Contents

Preface

The theme of 'identity' has been central to the development of the discipline of psychology, and advice about how to protect and strengthen individual 'identity' has been a powerful influence on a range of professional practices outside the discipline. There has been an underlying assumption made by psychologists and those who draw on psychological ideas, including in social work, that those who do not have strong identities are 'vulnerable', and that they desperately need their identity validated through some kind of 'recognition' given to them by their communities or by a trained professional. Ken McLaughlin, who has a background in critical debates in social work, dismantles that underlying assumption, showing how it leads to the disempowerment of the very people it is supposed to help. And he goes further, offering a critique of the way 'survivors' of different kinds are invited by psychologists and other professionals who draw on psychological ideas to configure themselves as victims in order to be able to claim access to services and to be valued as having the right kind of identity.

There are lessons here for all those in the caring professions who are concerned with the effects of psychology on their everyday practice, and there are, then, as a consequence, lessons for psychologists themselves. The book forces us to rethink what we are doing, and to reflect on the malign consequences of using identity as the touchstone of work with people who have been through difficult life-changing events.

This book series is designed to engage with developments in 'critical psychology' as it is understood by academic and professional psychologists and with the place of psychology in everyday commonsense understood as a process of psychologization. The key aim of the series is therefore to bring resources that are just outside psychology but which touch upon the concerns of psychologists, and to make explicit why an appreciation of these resources is necessary now to critical perspectives in the discipline. The phrase 'outwith psychology' captures this liminal character of the issues the authors address, and the different books explore debates at the edges of psychology; those outwith the discipline, those outwith existing conceptual frames, those outwith methodological approaches, those outwith national boundaries and those outwith the cultural phenomena that sustain or challenge mainstream psychology.

So, in this book, *Surviving Identity: Vulnerability and the Psychology of Recognition*, Ken McLaughlin gives us critical resources to be able to move into a realm 'outwith' identity. They are valuable resources for those who are survivors of psychology, whether we are still inside it or working to dismantle psychological concepts outside the discipline.

Ian Parker
Discourse Unit
Manchester Metropolitan University

Acknowledgements

I would like to thank Ian Parker, series editor, for encouraging me to write this book and also for his advice and encouragement at various stages during the course of its production. Thanks also to Kathryn Ecclestone, Phil Hodgkiss and Hilary Salt for reading and providing valuable feedback on the book in draft form; to Barbara Tisdall and Chris Yianni for comments on Chapter Four, and to Ann McLaughlin for her proofreading of various parts of the book as it progressed.

For Kieran and Lucy – and a life worth living, not just surviving

Introduction

Growing up in Scotland in the 1970s it was not uncommon during a visit to a town or city centre to see rather eccentric looking men wearing sandwich-boards proclaiming that 'The End is Nigh' and railing against such things as sin, gluttony and sloth. Most people either ignored them or gave them a pitying look; very few took them seriously. Forty years later such individuals may still be considered eccentric but their overall outlook of impending catastrophe and doomsday scenario is echoed by mainstream politicians, political activists and social commentators alike.

'The End is Nigh' could sum up the consensus of the contemporary period, which seems to be one of impending doom. Environmentalists inform us that we must curb our greed and reduce our carbon footprint to prevent global warming and resultant catastrophe. Rising global temperatures, we are told, could lead to an increase in diseases such as malaria and dengue fever. Scientific developments that in another era may have been heralded as giving humankind control over nature are charged with contributing to the current apocalyptic situation. Such things as genetically modified crops, rather than being seen as a potential answer to hunger and famine, are viewed by many as meddling with nature, distorting the food chain and potentially corrupting our genetic makeup. The industrialization of countries such as China, rather than being seen as a positive development that will raise the living standards of millions of people, is often looked on with horror due to the impact on the environment of such social development. Similarly, population growth, rather than being viewed positively, is perceived by many to be a regressive development with adverse implications for social space and a drain on the planet's resources. Such neo-Malthussians view people more as a consuming, destructive contaminant rather than as creative solvers of societal problems. From such perspectives it is our very survival that is at stake.

This political and cultural emphasis on survival resonates with much contemporary social policy which is increasingly directed at helping us survive the latest deadly disease, such as necrotizing fasciitis, AIDS, avian flu and swine flu, and also at keeping us healthy, both physically and mentally, once such mortal threats have been overcome. At first glance such a move seems progressive, but the continual drive to achieve 'health' may actually mask a degradation of what it means to be human, reducing us to biological beings whose main reason for living is to stay alive. The sandwich-board wearing eccentric railing against sin, gluttony and sloth has gone mainstream, only now in the guise of a health professional campaigning around such issues as obesity, smoking, alcohol consumption and sex (Fitzpatrick 2001).

The plethora of risks we are purported to face can make the very act of survival appear an achievement. Indeed, an increasing number of individuals are self-identifying as survivors of one thing or another. Survivors of the Nazi Holocaust, domestic violence and the psychiatric system have been joined by, among others, verbal abuse survivors, ex-gay survivors (who have survived attempts to cure them of their homosexuality – to make them 'ex-gay') and cult survivors. There have even been fake survivors, people who have been exposed as fabricating their memoirs of past abuse and recovery. Such is the popularity of the term that even critics of the prevailing therapeutic culture offer to show us 'How to *survive* without psychotherapy' (Smail 1996, my emphasis).

This growth of what some term a 'survivalist outlook' in western society is the subject of this book, with the main focus being on developments in the UK and, albeit to a lesser extent, the USA. Given that such a development has not arisen in a social vacuum, of particular interest is the link between broader social and political change and the rise of the concept and identity of the 'survivor'. As such, the 'survivor' will be considered not only from an individual perspective, as in those who would identify themselves as, for example, a 'sexual abuse survivor' or 'psychiatric survivor', but who do not see such an identity in collective terms, but also from the perspective of those for whom the embrace of the survivor identity also aligns them with a political collective with the aim of achieving social change.

In this respect, a key focus of analysis is on both individual and group identity. The subject of identity and what form of identification we are either ascribed or choose has taken on great significance in contemporary social and political life. Myriad social encounters, from applying for a job, academic or local authority grant, research questionnaire or health-related procedure will contain a form which asks you to identify yourself in relation to ethnicity, gender, disability and, in some cases, your sexuality. Similarly, many people will claim a variety of identities depending on social context, for example when referring to themselves as a 'professional, mother, partner, carer' etc. This ability to choose from a selection of different identities is limited for some people, who may find a stigmatized, devalued identity imposed on them from which it is not so easy to escape. Nevertheless, there is also an increasing tendency for individuals and groups to celebrate aspects of their identity (for example Gay Pride and Mad Pride in relation to sexuality and madness respectively), and while this can be done in order to combat the negative stereotypes attributed to the given identity, it also runs the risk of reifying it, of seeing it as a 'thing' rather than what it really is, namely a social and cultural construct. In such instances the identity can be both conservative and imprisoning, its very reproduction requiring continual social recognition that can, in effect, negate the possibility of the transcendence of identity.

The way specific individuals and groups identify themselves, then, is of major importance in a sociological and political sense, and also in terms of an individual's sense of self, both privately and in his or her engagement with others. In charting the changing nature of such identification it is therefore necessary to engage with the way in which demands around identity are articulated, the way various groups form together with specific beliefs and goals, and also the way in which such developments have been understood theoretically and historically.

However, in and of itself, this is insufficient in locating the significant influences on contemporary subject identification. It is also necessary to locate other pertinent societal developments which have a significant bearing on how dissent is articulated, internalized and expressed for public consumption. In order to do this the book will, at times, move from the specifics of social movement theory and formation to some perhaps less obvious influences on contemporary subjectivity, such as a climate of fear and mistrust within society and the concomitant promotion and internalization of a sense of individual and societal vulnerability. The structure of the book reflects this need to be both specific and general, aiming to link them together as each chapter develops in such a way as to inform our understanding of the identity debate in general and that of the survivor identity in particular. It is therefore important to look at areas of political action and social policy formation in such a way as to identify the more subtle ways a survivalist outlook permeates today's culture and which can become embedded within individual and collective consciousness. In order to do this the book covers three interlinked areas. The first two chapters analyse social movements and the ways in which they have come to focus on issues of cultural identity and the demand for recognition. The following two chapters look at the way in which the concept of 'the survivor' and the experience and articulation of 'trauma' began to be expanded to a wider array of human experiences which could also be 'survived', a move that was, as we shall see, itself influenced by changes in aspects of social movement formation, theory and practice, in particular its embracement of the concept of the vulnerable self. The final two chapters broaden the discussion by looking at the way the emphasis on survival and trauma has developed alongside, and indeed been coterminous with, a culture where psychological and therapeutic explanations for ever more aspects of life have proliferated, and where, as a result, the fragile and traumatized self is seen as axiomatic today.

As will be shown, such a vulnerable identity is, in many respects, cultivated by government, which not only plays a part in constructing individuals as such but also then implements policies with the ostensible aim of protecting such a fragile and at risk population. It is therefore necessary to highlight aspects of social policy that relate to this and the implications that follow from them. It is argued that the concept of 'survival' from myriad threats is deeply embedded within contemporary society to such an extent that it is not only those who identify as a survivor, but also all of us who are seen as surviving life and the daily interactions of which it is composed.

The way in which people have understood their sense of self-identity and group affiliation is subject to change. In Chapter 1 aspects of identity are considered but the focus is on group identity, on social movements, the influences on their formation and the way in which they have articulated their demands. Recent decades have seen the relative decline of the old mass movements that primarily organized around class and labour, and whose primary focus was on material inequality and the redistribution of power and wealth, to smaller movements more concerned with issues of cultural recognition and respect for social difference and diversity. This changing shape of social movements from the 'old' to the 'new' entails not only a change of focus but also a theoretical challenge to those who once espoused the primacy of class struggle as a political goal; in a postmodern world disenchanted with 'grand narratives', class becomes just one aspect of identity no more important than any other. As issues concerning race, gender, sexuality and disability have gained in prominence, that of class has faded, and, for many, is seen as less relevant today than other identities. Indeed it is possible to argue that the diminution of class identification and struggle was a prerequisite for the emergence of these other groups from the margins to the mainstream of political and cultural life.

However, the issue is not as clear cut as the above would suggest. The older class-focused movements and the new more culturally oriented ones were not always diametrically opposed; many social movement theorists and activists attempted to blend elements of some, if not all, aspects of identity-based injustice within a class paradigm as they tried to achieve a fairer, more equal society. Nevertheless, there was a discernible move towards the priority of culture and the positive affirmation of identity, from concerns over economic inequality to those of cultural recognition.

It is this political and cultural move from redistribution to recognition that is discussed in Chapter 2. Following a brief discussion of the intersection between personal and group identity and wider social change, the move within social movement theory and practice from a primary concern with material inequality to one in which the main aim was to redress issues of cultural injustice is the focus of analysis, with particular emphasis on the way in which a psychological form of both personal and group recognition is often demanded today. The debate ignited by Fraser's (1995) contribution to the dilemmas of justice in a 'post-socialist age' is discussed, with the contributions from a number of Fraser's critics utilized to highlight the many issues and complexities around contemporary political and cultural identification. This necessarily entails an engagement with poststructuralism and notions of subjectivity. However, to improve our understanding as to why 'survival' has become a motif for many individuals and groups in their quest for recognition and justice, it is necessary to look at how such 'abstract' theoretical concerns are themselves shaped by, and in turn shape, expressions of dissent and the articulation of identity.

Chapter 3 therefore looks at the subject of psychological trauma and how this influenced the rise of the 'survivor' as a paradigm of contemporary subject identification. Initially used almost exclusively with reference to the Holocaust, the concept then expanded although it still tended to refer to those who had suffered extreme experiences. This is no longer the case. Since the mid 1970s onwards, there has been a proliferation of those things that people are said to have 'survived'. The pain of trauma, whether real or imagined, is increasingly the prism through which claims for justice and recognition, whether group or individual in nature, are expressed. This chapter locates these developments with particular emphasis on the children of Holocaust survivors, the so called 'second-generation survivors' and their experience of transgenerational trauma. Also of significance is the influence of a therapeutically oriented form of feminism that accorded priority to the psychological harm experienced by women as a result of trauma, largely, though not exclusively, as a result of unequal gender relations and the abuse of power by men.

The experience of trauma, while it is felt in the present, is more concerned with the past. The survivors of trauma are often engaged in a battle for the past, concerned with 'speaking out', with 'breaking the silence' over some hitherto unacknowledged crime or trauma-inducing act. The self must be validated by the bestowal of belief on their account, acknowledgement of their feelings and the circumstances from which they have emerged; in other words there is a demand for recognition. The expansion of the concept of post-traumatic stress disorder (PTSD) is emblematic of the trend to emphasize trauma. First included in the American Psychiatric Association's *Diagnostic and Statistical Manual* as recently as 1980, the idea of 'trauma' has now gone mainstream; no longer confined to the clinic, it has permeated popular culture, including everyday conversations whether in a social, work or home setting.

This development entails the presentation of the self as injured, as psychologically damaged, albeit one that has 'survived', and is now able to speak out and in the process claim redress and recognition. However, by using insights from Foucault on the power of the confessional and drawing on dominant discursive repertoires in which to situate the self, the book suggests that such 'speaking out' necessitates a subject position that presents as inherently fragile, drawing as it does on a notion of the self as one that is perpetually traumatized.

The interaction of material changes within society and changing forms of social movement formation, campaigning and articulation towards an emphasis on psychological hurt is further illustrated in Chapter 4, which looks at how these developments have affected those categorized within a medical framework of mental disorder; psychiatric patients. Analysis of the forms of protest utilized by the opponents of psychiatry illustrate the influence of society on those movements. For example, early patients' organizations developed a critique of their oppression through a class-based analysis. Later, the influence of the politics of recognition and of 'speaking out' via testimonials is evident. Psychiatry's critics have also influenced wider perceptions of trauma by blurring the boundary between madness and sanity, questioning the evidence base of mainstream psychiatry, and bringing to the fore questions of autonomy and citizenship in relation to mental health legislation and psychiatric practice.

If the move within social movements is around recognition of trauma, and this relates to the increase of a subject positioning as a survivor, it is necessary to look again at the wider social context in which it has taken place, in particular the dominance of a therapeutic discourse and therapeutic identification. This is the subject of Chapter 5, which further explores the emphasis of the 'new social movements' on demands for recognition by detailing how such demands are increasingly focused on psychological damage to the fragile self, a process that saw therapeutic understandings proliferate by way of explanation and cure for an array of societal ills. This chapter explores the reasons behind this therapeutic transference from the clinic to the broader culture, discussing various explanations given for its rise to cultural prominence. Critiques that focus on the role of the psychiatry and psychology industries are discussed, as are those that implicate the pharmaceutical companies for creating new illnesses, which they then profess to be able to cure by the administration of the correct medication. Useful as these critiques are, it is argued that it is mistaken to reify them to the extent that they are viewed as omniscient powers controlling the mindset of the masses. To do so is to view people as gullible objects into which such ideas can simply be poured unmediated by other developments in society. As such, consideration is given to the way some social movements emphasize psychological weakness, undermine resilience and also the way in which the sick role and notions of health, illness, disability and 'madness' have been contested in recent years.

Within social policy there has been a move to institutionalize the concept of vulnerability, a move that can be aptly demonstrated by looking at the changing legal definitions of a 'vulnerable adult', which in a short space of time changed from one which seemed to envisage the 'vulnerable adult' as the exception, to one where a significant section of the population at any one time can be considered 'vulnerable'. Chapter 6 locates the above developments in relation to more material changes in society. As the old class-based movements lost both power and relevance within British society, to be replaced by the postmodern fragmentation of identity and solidarity, trade unions began to change their focus from one that emphasized the collective strength of the workforce to one that emphasized their psychological fragility.

With the working class no longer existing as a major power in contemporary political life, the search for new ways of negotiating workplace conflict and alienation drew on a newer, more socially acceptable mode of understanding, that of psychological vulnerability. Workplace disputes and tensions began to be discussed more and more in terms such as 'stress', often due to bullying and/or harassment from either bosses or colleagues. The coalescence of virtually all political players around the toxicity of interpersonal interaction and the promulgation of a politics of fear also forms the backdrop in our understanding of the reasons behind the rise of the concept of survival as a badge of pride.

The conclusion draws together the key themes of the book, noting the positive developments that have been achieved by many individual and social movement activists through their use of the politics of recognition, the trauma paradigm and the use of the survivor suffix. However, by locating these developments within a historical framework, such concepts need not be reified but seen as social, cultural and political constructs. To highlight their inadequacies and inherent contradictions is not to cast a slight on the integrity of the self, on the contrary it is an attempt to free the self from the imprisonment of the past as it is manifested in the present.

Shelter

E19-EDINBURGH Dalry
27, Dalry Road
Edinburgh
EH11 2BQ
Telephone: 0131 346 2468

You Were Served By 5815
On Till 1 at 13:14:47 on 8/04/2016

Product Details	Quantity	Total
Softback	1	3.00
Sub Total	1	3.00

Emboss Rcpt No:1443
MID:XXX54633   TID:XXXX1618
AID:A0000000031010
VISA DEBIT
XXXX XXXX XXXX 4910
N SEQ NO. : 00

                    GBP3.00
                    GBP3.00

BIT MY ACCOUNT
ED

THIS RECEIPT FOR YOUR

                                3.00

10008969

PAY
ICC
SALE
TOTAL
PLEASE D
PIN VERIF
PLEASE KEEP
RECORDS
AUTH CODE: 000

MAESTRO Tendere
Change
Receipt No:8969

7 8 6 2 9 0 7 9 0 0

1 Social movements old and new

In order to identify some of the social dynamics that have shaped contemporary forms of individual and group protest, and also to illustrate how many contemporary problems and demands are understood and articulated, it is first necessary to look at what is understood by the term 'social movement' and the factors that influence or inhibit their formation, success or failure, expansion or decline. In addition, it is necessary to provide some historical understanding to the present expressions of dissent and alienation. My intention is not to give a detailed analysis of social movement theory since this has been extensively done elsewhere (e.g. Tarrow 1994; Crossley 2002a; Snow et al. 2007a). Instead, I aim to provide an overview within which to situate the overall discussion of the way in which contemporary social problems are both articulated and contested.

Detailing some commonalities and contradictions within social movement theory and practice in historical context will highlight both changes and continuities within both theory and practice. This will also provide an account of the influences on the newer social movements in general, and survivor movements in particular. In so doing, it will become clear that it is not possible to pigeonhole any social movement within a given paradigm. Few, if any, movements are homogenous groups with no internal disagreements over either the exact problem they confront or the tactics with which to do so. At times, it is those who share the same general view of the problem who differ the most in how best to tackle it, as illustrated by the numerous splits and further fragmentations within the radical left of the second half of the twentieth century.

The same is true of those organizations that purport to carry the radical banner today. The 'environmental movement', for example, contains a variety of groups with very different aims; from those solely concerned with small-scale local neighbourhood issues to those who harbour revolutionary goals, others will sit somewhere between the extremes while some will traverse various groups at various times. Nevertheless, it is possible to identify some current trends and locate some of the factors in their creation that are of central importance in locating the roots of the survivor identity that will be discussed in later chapters.

First, I wish to look at some definitions of social movements and the problems with providing a precise universal analytic category. Second, I look at some theoretical attempts to make sense of social movements and how these have changed historically, specifically related to the changing repertoires of the new social movements (many of which are now quite old). Third, I wish to highlight a trend whereby there is an implicit contempt for the masses contained within an increasingly middle class dominated social movement sphere.

Defining social movements

Defining the criteria necessary for a collection of people to constitute a social movement is not as straightforward as it can first appear. At its most basic, Giddens (1997: 511) defines a social movement as a 'collective attempt to further a common interest or secure a common goal, through collective action outside the sphere of established institutions'. The first problem with such a definition is that it does not tell us how many people are necessary before a group becomes a collective. Is it two, twenty, one hundred, ten thousand? Do they share a united, clear goal or a disparate set of linked goals? The numerical question is also a historical one as definitions are shaped by the circumstances in which they are produced. For example, Wilson defines a social movement as 'a conscious, collective, organized attempt to bring about or resist *large-scale* change in the social order by non-institutionalised means' (Wilson 1973: 8, my emphasis). This emphasis on large-scale change is reflective of the time of organized labour, feminism, gay politics and civil rights. Radical change was on the agenda with competing visions of how to organize society on offer. However, Wilson's quote also acknowledges that social movements may not be about achieving change; on the contrary many may be actively resisting change to defend the status quo.

An emphasis on large-scale change is still the main criterion for some writers today. However, more recent and detailed definitions have expanded to include not only large-scale social movements but also small, localized group formations, such as NIMBYs (not in my back yard) or other neighbourhood groups. So, for Abercrombie et al.

(2006: 358) 'the aims of social movements can be broad, as in the overthrow of existing government, or narrow, as in the installation of traffic calming measures'. This is instructive not just in the way the conceptualization of social movements has modified over the years. The narrowing of goals from large-scale change to campaigns over road safety does more than conflate the two; the juxtaposition of social revolution with pedestrian crossings also has the rhetorical effect of making the former look ridiculous, the latter reasonable and achievable.

Following a discussion of the pros and cons of a number of definitions, Snow et al. (2007b) favour the following conceptualization of social movements as being

> Collectivities acting with some degree of organization and continuity outside of institutional or organizational channels for the purpose of challenging or defending extant authority, whether it is institutionally or culturally based, in the group, organization, society, culture, or world order of which they are part.
>
> (Snow et al. 2007b: 11)

Snow et al. also differentiate between social movements and interest groups. While acknowledging that there can be many overlaps in terms of shared goals and objectives, they nevertheless see three crucial distinctions. First, interest groups are generally defined in relation to the government or polity, whereas social movements have connections to a much wider range of social institutions. Second, being generally embedded within the existing political sphere, interest groups tend to have some degree of political legitimacy; social movements, on the other hand, can be opposed to the existing polity and/or be in the process of attempting to achieve recognition as a political actor. Third, tactical differences are evident, with interest groups mainly using institutional means such as political lobbying, while the tactics of social movements can include demonstrations, boycotts, industrial action and sit ins. I purposefully avoided listing violence as a tactic specific to social movements. While it most certainly is a tactic at times, to list it solely as a potential attribute of social movements fails to acknowledge the use of violence by institutional bodies of the state such as the police and border control agencies. This runs the risk of pathologizing movement violence and both naturalizing and neutralizing state violence.

Even allowing for the many overlaps between social movements and interest groups, Snow et al. conclude that they are

not so much different species as members of the same species
positioned differently in relation to the polity or state. But that
differential positioning is sufficiently important to produce different sets of strategic and tactical behaviours, and thus different
kinds of collectivities.

(Snow et al. 2007b: 8)

The contention that social movements invariably lie outside the
sphere of established institutions, and also outside the state, reflects
the majority view that tends to view social movements as challenging
current views and practices condoned by those with institutional
power. Again though, things are not quite so clear cut. Many professionals work to destabilize institutional power at the same time as
being part of the institution. For example, the 'Radical Social Work'
movement's slogan of 'Both In and Against the State' embodied the
tactic of attempting to subvert the system from within. Similarly, the
loose umbrella of professionals given the collective rubric of 'anti-
psychiatry' in the 1960s contained many individuals who wielded
substantial institutional power, but who nevertheless attempted to use
this against traditional medical paradigms and practices. This tradition continues within both psychiatry and psychology (e.g. Thomas
1997; Parker 2007). It also chimes with Tarrow's claim that social
movements can be defined as collective challenges 'based on common
purposes and social solidarities in sustained interaction with elites,
opponents and authorities' (Tarrow 1998: 4). The emphasis on interaction does not negate working with or even within the organization
of social work, psychology or psychiatry for those respective activist-
professionals.

This brief discussion highlights the difficulty of finding a universal
definition of social movements and their aims and objectives. There is
no clear delineation between the constitutive parts of various social
movements in terms of numbers, tactics, goals, leadership, organization or non-organization. Nevertheless, it is possible to identify
specific social movements, albeit in the knowledge that we are at times
using heuristic models to conceptualize fluid entities. In similar vein, it
is possible to locate some of the factors in social movement formation.

Theorizing social movements

The theoretical focus on social movements has differed not only
historically but also geographically. Influenced by Marx and Hegel,
European scholars favoured an approach that looked at key

contradictions and conflicts in society and how they give rise to social movements that attempt to address them. In the USA, while the dialectical approach had some influence, there was more of a focus on a broader range of movements, with the aim of locating the empirical conditions that allowed or inhibited their emergence and 'much less concern to pin these movements to the dialectics of history or a specific type of society' (Crossley 2002a: 11).

My approach favours the historical-dialectical approach in that I am interested in exploring the way that societal conflicts and contradictions are articulated and discontent expressed. However, I wish to go beyond a class conflict analysis. While class is certainly an important social dynamic, class consciousness and class mobilization are no longer such powerful social forces as they were in the past. The decline of class consciousness and working class organization does not mean that the problems they confronted have gone away, but changes in both subjective and objective conditions influence their expression and articulation. It may be the case that much of the alienation and distress of modern society has a class base, but increasingly that is not how it is felt privately or expressed publicly.

Within the social movement literature, different theoretical positions provide various views of social actors and the movements that they make up. Whereas 'collective behaviour' theories tended to view social movements as irrational psychological responses, as 'mobs' exhibiting some form of collective hysteria, 'rational actor' theory sees individuals as pursuing specific goals to maximize gains and minimize losses or hardship. The latter approach was adapted from economics, particularly the cost-benefit analytic approach; it was not just individuals that were rational but movements also (McCarthy and Zald 1977).

Much early work on social movement formation focused on their emergence under conditions of expanding political opportunities. Making demands directly of the state, around such things as labour and civil rights, they were located within the political process. As such, 'political process theory' was arguably the dominant theoretical approach in the 1970s and into the 1980s (Goodwin and Jasper 2004). The latter decades of the twentieth century also saw increasing examination of the cultural side of social movements and, more recently, there has been greater interest in the role of emotions in protest (e.g. Tarrow 1994; Gould 2004).

As political opportunities open up, it makes it easier for people to join a social movement, and via their collective action they create new opportunities which can lead to the formation of other social movements. This begs the question of what exactly is a 'political opportunity'? For Tarrow, they are those 'dimensions of the political environment that provide incentives for people to take collective action by affecting their expectations for success or failure' (Tarrow 1994: 85). This would indicate an acknowledgement that political opportunities are not solely objective entities waiting to be discovered, but are things that are open to interpretation. The weighing up of whether the 'incentives' are worthwhile and meet 'expectations', implies a degree of subjective interpretation. With this in mind, it has been suggested that there is a need to abandon invariant theoretical models that attempt to subsume the complexity of social movements into a universal framework (Goodwin and Jasper 2004). There is also a need to recognize the way culture permeates not only social movement agents but also social movement theorists.

Social movements are often seen as being the political expression of public dissatisfaction with some aspect of societal relations, as giving political voice to disparate actors. An interesting rider to this, though, is given by Honneth (2003), who argues that this prioritization of small groups of social movements as being representative of demands for social justice and recognition ignores a multitude of other human injustice and discontent. In other words, certain forms of social injustice are moved to the centre of public political life, while others, what Honneth terms the pre-political, are downgraded or ignored. Honneth's work has proven influential and will be discussed further in Chapter 2.

It is commonly assumed that before there can be the formation of a social movement there has to be both grievance and strain. Put simply, there has to be something to oppose before there can arise an oppositional social movement. Such grievances do not in themselves create the conditions for mobilization; people often put up with abhorrent treatment without it leading to collective action. Strain, where opposition to these practices is voiced, is also necessary before such grievances are articulated (however inadequately) and collective mobilization achieved. In discussing the grievance/strain requirement, Crossley (2002a) points out that, while they are a prerequisite, they require at least five additional conditions to achieve social movement formation: movement culture; opportunities and the responses of agents of control; pre-existing networks; resources; and trigger events.

The culture of the movement is important as it has to agree, however tentatively and despite many possible disagreements and contradictions, a schematic that locates the grievances outside the individuals concerned. As Crossley (2002a: 146) puts it, if 'groups collectively attribute their misfortune to their own personal failings then they are unlikely to form an oppositional movement'. The existence of pre-existing networks can facilitate formation. If members already belong to one group they are more likely to be in a position to form another. Resources can also be crucial, for example to pay full-time activists an income and to hold meetings, provide transport to events and organize demonstrations, etc. Trigger events, which can encapsulate group anger about some aspect of policy and practice, can also prove influential in mobilizing oppositional forces. For example, the mental health user/survivor-led campaign group Mad Pride was formed, at least in part, in response to government proposals for more coercive mental health legislation in England during the late 1990s.

A 'trigger event' in itself does not necessarily lead to movement formation; this is dependent on a combination of the other factors. For example, the catalyst for the civil rights movement in the USA is often credited to Rosa Parks' refusal to give up her seat on a bus to a white man in the city of Montgomery, the capital of the state of Alabama. The subsequent furore and the boycott of the bus company by the black population is seen as a pivotal moment in race relations history. However, Rosa Parks was no downtrodden black woman who finally resisted discrimination on that eventful day. On the contrary, she was a seasoned activist who had made similar protests in the past which had generated little publicity or public outrage, far less a sophisticated campaign. Following her arrest on this occasion, the Black Church proved very effective in mobilizing its constituency, with Martin Luther King informing people that all the ministers in Montgomery fully endorsed the boycott plan and had promised to promote it to their congregations on Sunday at church (Morris 2004). Not only did the church endorse the boycott, thereby giving it legitimacy within the black population, but it also provided the emergent movement with essential resources such as the use of its extensive communication networks, organized congregations and vast financial and cultural assets.

The emotional power of religion, along with nationalism, is identified by Tarrow (1994) as a recurring factor in social movement mobilization due to its 'ready made' symbolism and rituals that can be utilized by movement leaders. It is in this regard that Morris (2004) is critical of those writers (e.g. Snow 1992) who contend that the central frame of the civil rights movement was one of 'rights'. While this was certainly an important aspect, it downplays the church's emphasis on respect and religion, which tapped into the emotional, cultural and material world of much of the black population in that locality at that time. The 'knowledge' that 'God was on their side' also helped motivate the congregation.

In attempting to move social movement theory forward, Crossley (2002a) incorporates the work of Pierre Bourdieu, specifically his concepts of 'field' and 'habitus', into his analysis of social movements. For Bourdieu the concept of the habitus is important because with it,

> you can refer to something that is close to what is suggested by habit, while differing from it in one important respect. The habitus, as the word implies, is that which one has acquired, but which has become durably incorporated in the body in the form of permanent dispositions.
>
> (Bourdieu 1993: 86)

In other words, the 'habitus' refers to the way in which social, cultural and moral codes are absorbed by social agents becoming embedded within them. This can involve linguistic schemas, 'appropriate' ways of behaving in various social contexts, cultural competence, belief systems, etc. However, this is not a culturally deterministic model but an agentic one; Bourdieu recognizes that we are active agents, our habitus may be formed but we also do the forming. As Crossley puts it:

> Human action does not emerge out of 'nothingness', for Bourdieu, but rather out of a habitus formed by way of the history of the agent. On the 'agentic' side this conception emphasizes that we make ourselves through our various ways of acting; our habits are a residue of our previous patterns of action. Nevertheless, we make ourselves in particular ways, in response to the conditions we find ourselves in, and this means that we are always 'something' rather than the pure 'nothingness' of the Sartrean schema, that is, we are always characterized by concrete preferences, schemas, dispositions, interests, know how, etc.
>
> (Crossley 2002a: 172)

If the notion of the habitus has echoes of the 'framing theorists', who sought to analyse the way social movements framed their problems and demands, it surpasses them by specifically linking habitus and fields to the structural and material conditions that affect identified social groups and classes. It therefore raises the issue of the material circumstances by which different groups have inculcated differing habitus, and advances a strong theory of symbolic power and of the way in which some issues are given more political credence than others (Crossley 2002a).

Bourdieu's work sought to unify various dichotomies such as the subjective and the objective, structure and agency. He emphasized that it is the relation between them that is of most importance. Habitus is therefore 'the dialectic of the internalization of externality and the externalization of internality' (Bourdieu 1977: 72). For Bourdieu, society is not a whole system but rather is constituted by myriad networks of objective relations structured in social space, which he terms 'fields'. The differentiation of fields is objective in that we occupy various network positions in social space depending on the resources we possess. However, we also act on the fields subjectively; in other words we internalize the social structure but we can also act upon it. Bourdieu recognizes that we are embodied beings but also that we can and do make choices, albeit ones which are shaped by the social structure in general and specific field in particular. He conjoins the reflexivity and cognition inherent within ethnomethodology while simultaneously situating the individual within the wider social structure. We are socialized subjects who exhibit 'socialized subjectivity' (Bourdieu and Wacquant 1992: 127).

The resources that agents possess are what Bourdieu refers to as 'capital', which he breaks down into various components; economic capital (money, possessions, property, etc.), cultural capital (educational and professional qualifications, cultural etiquette), symbolic capital (status, prestige) and social capital (connections, networks, etc). All these types of capital can help or hinder the agent depending on the specific field; for example, a professional social work qualification carries more capital within the field of social work than in the ranks of professional football. It is also important to recognize that such cultural resources are held in differing quantities by different social groups, which in turn affects their life chances, their way of seeing and knowing the world and their place within it.

In addition, one field can impact upon another in ways that can generate strains and grievances. Through analysing the interaction of fields, Bourdieu provides a much sharper analytical framework through which to understand the broader structural trends influencing social movement formation and the strategies that are open to those movements. In the psychiatric field for example, the options for protest available to patients locked up in the old asylum system were far fewer than are available today (Crossley 2002b).

The insights afforded by Crossley are extremely instructive in understanding contemporary expressions of distress, alienation and grievance. They allow us to look at the wider social structure and how it impacts on the various fields that social actors inhabit. As his example of psychiatry shows, options for protest can change as fields open or close. This shows the need to identify the factors behind the opening up, and, just as importantly, the closing off, of options that have influenced the rise in identity politics in general, and specifically the related trend for people to identify as a 'survivor'. This necessitates attention to the historical emergence of the discourses and meaning through which contemporary views of social and individual problems are articulated. As new 'regimes of truth' (Foucault 1980) are established it is necessary to see how they have influenced contemporary social movements.

Repertoires of recognition

Tilly (1995) has observed that the form of protest utilized by social agents changes according to socio-historical and geographical circumstances. The choice of action, what he terms *repertoires*, is therefore a learned cultural creation. As he notes,

> People learn to break windows in protest, attack pilloried prisoners, tear down dishonored houses, stage public marches, petition, hold formal meetings, organize special interest associations. At any particular point in history, however, they learn only a rather small number of alternative ways to act collectively.
> (Tilly 1995: 26)[1]

The point Tilly is making is that there is a vast array of repertoires or tactical measures that can be utilized, but, due to the specific circumstances of the day, only a very limited few are. It implies not only that choices are constrained by circumstances but also that people can affect change.

There are myriad social movements which employ a variety of repertoires today, from bombings and shootings, riots and other civil disturbance, direct action, engagement with the authorities, awareness raising, local neighbourhood initiatives through to more macro concerns, to name but a few. Some movements will employ a range simultaneously and some may have some members who will abide by the law, while others in the group will have little compunction over breaking it. Also, in conjunction with the socio-historical mode of protest within a socially stratified society, various actors will have access to different resources. For example, within the labour movement, the ability to withdraw labour by going on strike has, for some time, been seen as a key repertoire for workers. However, such action is not available to the millions of unemployed.[2] It is not possible to withdraw labour if you do not have any to withdraw. Therefore, understanding the processes behind the choice of action taken at any given period is important. It is never strictly causal in the sense that A causes B, it is always complex and multifactoral; people do not respond to a given stimulus like animals in a laboratory.

The above point is useful in reminding us that the particular form of protest is always linked to the resources available to social actors, and that we need to be careful not to subsume lots of particular group circumstances under an overarching theory of contemporary social action. Nevertheless, it is possible to identify some broad societal trends that shape the way both individual and social concerns are expressed today. Of significance is the way that a dominant and recurring contemporary repertoire is around the motif of recognition, whereby there is a demand for a specific social group or identity to be accorded positive cultural respect. This has been a particular feature of what have been termed the 'new social movements'.

New Social Movements

In post-industrial societies the emergence of new social movements (NSMs) gained momentum from the 1970s onwards, influenced, at least in part, by the failure of the social protests of 1968 that many participants hoped would awaken the revolutionary class consciousness that would lead to proletarian revolution. These new movements differed from their class-based predecessors in terms of ideology, origins, structure and goals. For Habermas (1981, 1987), this meant a move away from the old 'capital versus labour' struggles characteristic of the Labour movement, which focused almost exclusively on pay and working conditions, towards campaigns and disputes arising from what he termed the 'colonization of the lifeworld'. The labour movement, in Habermas's view, had become integrated into the system/state to such an extent that it no longer constituted a radical agent of change.

Demands around purely monetary gain are instrumental in nature and easily placated by financial reward. In Britain, for example, the Labour party and the trade unions in effect helped integrate the working class into the machinery of British capitalism. From this perspective, the truly radical movements are those concerned with wider issues around identity and our place in the world, our relations to others and the ways in which we live our lives. Non-conformity and the challenges posed to accepted ways of doing things, then, come not from organized labour, but from movements such as feminism, environmentalism, lesbian and gay groups and others advocating a different set of societal values and an alternative way of living.

The new social movements also emphasized the politics of difference. For Swingewood (2000: 236) this meant that, 'the subjugated and the marginal, those whose voices had been drowned by the dominant discourses or simply forgotten, were rehabilitated sociologically and historically to engage in dialogue between the past, the present and the future'. It went further than this. Groups also came to prominence that campaigned not only for those whose voices had been silenced but also for those without voices – animals, the planet, future generations. While many of these groups proclaim to embrace radical change, their position would not sit unfavourably with that of the eighteenth century defender of tradition and conservative philosopher Edmund Burke's belief that, 'Society is indeed a contract . . . [it is] a partnership not only between those who are living, but between those who are living, those who are dead and those who are to be born' (Burke 1993 [1790]: 96).

In purporting to speak for animals, the planet or the unborn such activists effectively give themselves carte-blanche to propose whatever they like; without a mandate from their 'constituency', animals being dumb, the planet a rock, and the unborn being just that, it is not possible to know what they want. Speaking on their behalf becomes a rhetorical device to lend some credence to *the speaker's* favoured course of human action in the present.

Contemporary conflicts, then, are not predominantly class based or necessarily located where the interests of capital and labour clash, but rather occur 'at the seam between system and lifeworld' (Habermas 1981: 36). The lifeworld, that area of daily interaction with others, is increasingly being colonized by a system of commodification and instrumental rationality. For example, Klein (2000) points out how public space is increasingly colonized by corporate advertising via the ubiquity of billboards and hoardings, shopping malls and other consumer outlets to such an extent that commercial messages are virtually the only ones permitted. The new social movements challenge this through such things as campaigns to protect the environment from the effects of economic expansion, as in the protests against the building of additional airport terminals or roads.

Likewise, the expansion of welfare systems into family life impacts on the way relationships are negotiated on a micro level and reconfigures the terrain where disputes take place. The question becomes not one of compensations that the welfare state can provide. Rather, the question is how to defend or reinstate endangered lifestyles, or how to put reformed lifestyles into practice. In short, the new conflicts are not sparked by *problems of distribution*, but concern *the grammar of forms of life*.

(Habermas 1981: 33, emphasis in original)

The salient point here is that change is not wholly confined to the level of the cultural or the symbolic; it can also include self-change.

Several critics of Habermas accuse him of exaggerating the extent to which class conflict has declined, claiming that while he improves our understanding of many aspects of contemporary society and social theory, it is not the case that there is a fundamentally new relationship between the old and new social movements. They claim that he has consigned the old labour disputes to the dustbin too readily. For example, Edwards (2004) uses the examples of 'anti-corporatism', 'community unionism' and the British firefighters' dispute of 2002–03 to claim that issues of working conditions and wage disputes have resurfaced within many contemporary social movements. According to Edwards, some campaigns, such as that for a Living Wage, are more accurately described as a combination of Habermas's old and new politics:

In Living Wage campaigns we see the 'old' concerns of material distribution, minimum wages and rights at work encased within language and action more easily identifiable as Habermas' 'new' politics. Work-related demands are couched in community-based claims surrounding the quality of life, basic human rights, inclusivity and participation. Here, however, they are not new political conflicts *per se*, but rather new ways of communicating 'old' struggles.

(Edwards 2004: 122)

In attempting to resuscitate the labour movement by the use of such an example, Edwards risks underestimating the decline of working class politics. It is certainly the case that workplace disputes will, from time to time, lead to industrial action. However, in looking for such examples, it needs to be borne in mind that, not so long ago, there was little need to look very far; industrial disputes were common, bitter, often violent, and prolonged. The very fact of having to look merely demonstrates the extent of the change. He does have a point, though, in that the way in which work-related concerns are expressed today differs from the past, something that is discussed in more detail in subsequent chapters.

Others also insist that there are elements of the old and the new within the demands of specific movements. Several disability activists point out that the disability movement, while commonly termed a 'new' movement, also campaigns around 'old' issues such as material (re)distribution and rights of citizenship (e.g. Shakespeare 1993). Shakespeare also makes the point that many black and women's groups also straddle the old/new dichotomy, campaigning around issues of political rights and power and also around lifestyle or cultural rights.

Such an empirically focused debate over which aspects of both the old and new social movements contain similar repertoires and tactics, while interesting, tends to miss the point. As Crossley (2002a) points out, it is the paradigm shift in how the working class is viewed, and also views itself, that is of historical importance. For the old movements the working class were the main social movement in capitalist society. For the NSMs they are but one identity that should not be accorded any special status. NSMs then analyse society to identify

> other schisms, conflicts and movements *at the heart of the modern social order* . . . The thesis of NSMs, in this respect, is a thesis about the shift in the mode of historicity in western societies and the corresponding shift in the central struggle of those societies. It is this mode of historicity and its faultlines which lends NSMs their 'newness', rather than any particular empirical feature of those movements.
>
> (Crossley 2002a: 151, emphasis in original)

It is certainly possible to trace aspects of identity and cultural politics in the old labour-based social movements. However, NSM theory has brought that aspect of political, or sub-political, life to the fore and, in the process, sidelined the traditional class-based focus on party formation, the role of the state and revolution. For many NSMs it is the state that is seen as the medium through which all societal disputes can be resolved. This contemporary return to Hegel has the effect of allowing the relationship between the state and citizen to be reformulated; the former is now recast as a benign arbiter between competing identity claims, the latter as dependent on state beneficence.

This can be seen in Williams' (1999) view that the rise of consumer-led groups has contributed to the emergence of an active welfare subject as opposed to a passive recipient of welfare. Williams (1999) favours a radical pluralist notion of democracy. This, according to her, allows for a *politics of differentiated universalism* to emerge which will allow the management of competing group claims. However, the active welfare subject is still a welfare rather than an autonomous subject. The management of competing group claims also increasingly falls to the state and its proxies, and has also influenced a trend whereby other people are viewed as the problem and the state as the solution (McLaughlin 2008). This not only risks individualizing social problems but also gives the authorities more control over the lifeworld. A viewpoint that sees people as inherently problematic gives rise to profoundly anti-human and authoritarian sentiments, and, as is shown below, this is indeed a feature propagated by many contemporary social movements and political commentators.

Moving against the masses

The focus of social movement theory has tended to be on the collective efforts of the oppressed and marginalized in society. McAdam (1982) defined social movements as 'those organized efforts on the part of *excluded* groups, to promote or resist changes in the structure of society that involve recourse to noninstitutional forms of political participation' (McAdam 1982: 25, my emphasis). Even when the theoretical gaze moved towards those termed NSMs, for some this aspect remained a prerequisite. According to Oliver (1996), NSMs are seen to contain four essential elements: they remain on the margins of the political system; they offer a critical evaluation of society; they imply a society with different forms of valuation and distribution; and the issues they raise transcend national boundaries. Such analyses do not necessarily correspond adequately to today's situation. Many contemporary social movements and many of their leading activists are not on the margins of the political system; on the contrary they are very much a part of it. Their critique of society is limited and partisan, their forms of valuation and distribution are one-sided and they can be used to bolster rather than transcend national boundaries.

The case of environmentalism provides the clearest illustration of this contradiction. Far from being marginalized, many leading figures in environmental politics are either middle class or part of the establishment (Knight 2008). So, while many NSM advocates see their increasing political representation and influence as progressive democracy in action, it could be argued instead that, rather than a triumph of democracy, there has been a removal of the working class and concomitant middle class colonization of the political sphere. As such they can be very conservative in nature. As Offe (1987: 75) notes, they 'often strongly emphasize the preservation of traditional communities, identities and social as well as cultural environments'.

Similarly, Cotgrove and Duff (2003) argue that much environmentalism represents a challenge to the dominant beliefs of modernity. They note that many of its adherents do not share the modern age's belief in the benefits of science and technology, are sceptical over the 'efficacy' of the capitalist market economy and its emphasis on economic growth and profit, and are against what they see as the usurpation of the policy decision-making process by experts. As such, they see environmentalism as a 'challenge to the hegemonic ideology which legitimates the institutions and politics of industrial capitalism' (Cotgrove and Duff 2003: 77). However, attitudes to science within environmentalism are ambivalent; many environmentalists may be anti-science in that they lack belief in science's ability to solve contemporary social problems, but much of the environmental argument is based on the premise that 'The Science' offers irrefutable evidence to substantiate their views on the correct response to such things as climate change and rising sea levels. In effect, rather than surpassing the 'usurpation of the political policy decision making by experts', environmentalism merely insists on replacing the current experts with its own, those with relevant PhDs or other experts who hold mainstream environmentalist views on what the problem is and what is required to rectify it (Heartfield 2009).

Of importance in understanding these developments is to recognize a key feature of contemporary western society: the evacuation of the masses from the political sphere. The decline of the labour movement and working class consciousness during the latter decades of the twentieth century has created a vacuum between the masses and the political establishment and, at least in part, explains the domination of the current public political sphere by middle and elite constituencies. Today, for example, many MPs will be career politicians with little connection to the electorate. The Left, disorganized and weakened by the setbacks of the 1970s and 1980s, exemplified by the defeat of the 1984–85 miners' strike and various pieces of anti-trade union legislation, has also been ideologically weakened following the collapse of the Soviet bloc. As a consequence it has had to rethink tactics and strategies. For many activists there was an embracement of green politics in an effort to refocus the political agenda and regain some political authority.

In the process there has also been a shift in what is defined as radical or progressive politics today. For some, to be radical today means turning conventional radicalism on its head. Consider this rallying cry from environmental campaigner George Monbiot, who is calling for 'a campaign not for abundance but for austerity. It is a campaign not for more freedom but for less. Strangest of all, it is a campaign not just against other people, but against ourselves' (Monbiot 2006: 215). The contradiction in such an approach is readily apparent. As Heartfield (2009: 50) argues, 'telling working class people that their greed is the problem is not an obvious route to popular support'. And if the masses cannot be persuaded to change their ways, then, for some, the only resort is repression. Monbiot (2008) sees 'resorting to totalitarianism' as a possible solution to the 'problem of capitalism'. According to Heartfield (2009: 46), 'what Monbiot means by the "problem of capitalism" is not the limits it puts on working-class living standards, but rather the growth in those living standards'. Compare Monbiot's view to that of the leading trade unionist Samuel Gompers, speaking in 1890, arguing that the whole labour movement could be summed up in one word, 'more': 'We do want more, and when it becomes more, we shall still want more. And we shall never cease to demand more until we have received the results of our labor' (quoted in Heartfield 2009: 45).

The call for austerity, to cut back, to live within our means was once the terrain of the right wing, being identified in the 1980s with the policies and ideology of the neo-conservatism of Margaret Thatcher in the UK and Ronald Reagan in the USA. However, such sentiments have been embraced by many 'radicals' today, so that when the UK Conservative-Liberal coalition government, which came to power in 2010, proposed widespread austerity measures, much of the criticism was over where the cuts should be made, rather than making arguments or campaigning for a defence of existing jobs and services. In this context, calls for 'more' are likely to be dismissed as being unrealistic in terms of the economy and also of being dangerous to the planet.

The campaign for 'less freedom' is also evident in many environmental campaigners' admiration of the totalitarian regime in China in respect of its enforcement of a one-child-only policy. Sir Richard Attenborough, patron of the Optimum Population Trust, a neo-Malthusian organization, is concerned about population growth and seeks to promote measures that would reduce the birth rate. He would like to see a planetary one-child policy. Some environmentalists, including an eco-feminist writing in the UK *Guardian* (Fitzgerald 2009), warn us that without such a policy in place the Chinese population would be approximately 400 million people higher today.

When you have a feminist in awe at a totalitarian state's control over women's reproductive rights, it is clear that the old political frameworks and identifications no longer have much meaning. The freedom for women to choose is still there, provided, of course, that they only choose, at most, one child.

Such middle class contempt for the masses is nothing new. Le Bon (1912) argued that crowds were motivated by instinct as opposed to reason and developed psychological theories concerned with the behaviour of the 'crowd'. The elites were held to be capable of suppressing instinct while the masses were not. Drawing on this work, Freud saw a clear parallel between the individual regressed psyche and the masses, the relationship between the ego and the id being replicated in the social world by that between the elites and the masses. In each case, the former is viewed as the rational controller, the latter as unruly and irrational and therefore in need of control by the mind, the state or the therapist.

Carey (1992), in an illuminating analysis of the work of early twentieth century writers and cultural commentators such as George Bernard Shaw, Ezra Pound, Virginia Woolf and Aldous Huxley, shows how the masses were viewed as semi-human swarms, with extermination a not unconsidered solution to the dangers to civilization posed by such 'promiscuous hordes'. Such sentiments are also evident today. Reading the website of the Optimum Population Trust, especially those articles expressing concern over the effects of immigration on the UK and the high birth rate in developing countries, there is a tangible sense that they regard such children as toxic agents harmful to the planet. The issues raised by such groups may transcend national borders, but national borders and anti-immigration controls are strengthened by calls for the nation to be saved from the 'threat' of over-population, whether from outside or within such borders.

An implicit contempt for the masses is not confined to environmental campaigners. Much of social policy and social work betrays a similar contempt for the masses. The changing focus of the radical social work movement in the 1970s and 1980s is indicative not only of this trend, but also of the move from the old class-focused struggle to the new campaigns around identity and culture. From viewing the working class as the agent of the revolutionary transformation of society, *as the solution*, within ten years activists came to see the same people as requiring professional training to eradicate their prejudices; in other words they were now seen *as the problem* (Langan 2002). In demonstrating their antiracist credentials, social work student practice often takes the form of admonishing a client for using inappropriate or offensive language (Collins et al. 2000). Indeed, for some, to be truly 'anti-oppressive', the social worker should intervene in any 'oppressive' conversation they hear, whether or not it is directed at them (Dominelli 2002). The example Dominelli (2002) gives is related to members of the public making derogatory remarks about asylum seekers and neatly encapsulates the way public authorities are seen as enlightened beings over the oppressive masses.

Such developments also illustrate how as personal interactions become politicized, state actions can be depoliticized (McLaughlin 2008). For example, social work now plays a key role in the internal regulation of immigration policy, social workers being obliged to inform the Home Office if a failed asylum seeker, or anyone else they consider to be in the UK unlawfully, tries to claim community care services. There is evidence that local authorities are interpreting in the narrowest possible way the 'eligibility criteria' for services that immigrants must satisfy. A Court of Appeal judge lambasted Leicester City Council, stating that its policies amounted to starving 'immigrants out of the country by withholding last resort assistance' (quoted in Humphries 2004: 105). In the topsy-turvy world of social work, this could lead to the social worker demonstrating their 'antiracist' credentials by admonishing the asylum seeker for using inappropriate language, while at the same time refusing them services because they are not considered 'one of us'.

Social policy provides further examples where seemingly benign proposals hide anti-human sentiments. Today, although few would subscribe to the radical feminist view that all heterosexual sex equates to rape, the idea that relationships are inherently abusive underpins many government initiatives, for example that health visitors should routinely ask pregnant women if they are experiencing domestic violence (Hehir 2004). Likewise, as we will discuss in detail in Chapter 6, the introduction of the Independent Safeguarding Authority's vetting and barring scheme for those working with children and vulnerable adults may be presented as necessary to protect the vulnerable, yet it also betrays contempt for carers, who are viewed as potential predators, and also expresses disdain for those it is intended to protect, by classing them all as 'vulnerable' people unable to exercise autonomy.

Conclusion

This chapter has provided an overview of some general trends within social movements themselves and of various attempts to theorize these developments. Of significance in the contemporary period is the decline of working class political organization, the collapse of the old left/right political ideologies, and a growing concern with cultural and lifestyle politics. This is not to look back nostalgically at some mythical golden age. Instead, it illustrates how this decline has helped to pave the way for the articulation and popularization of new social movements. They may have already existed in various forms but the vacuum created by the evacuation of the working class has allowed other groups to have their 'voices heard' (to use a favoured expression of the discourse).

One effect is that as some repertoires of contention become closed off, others open up and their space for manoeuvre increases. However, I have also sought to show that, in many instances, the rise of many such groups is not as democratic as it can first appear. The trend towards a political sphere dominated by the middle/upper class can find expression in a palpable disdain for the masses who do not share their cultural norms or political outlook. When establishment figures, whether in government or in campaign groups are so anti-mass consumption, critics such as Heartfield (2009) are perhaps correct in their view that such campaigners' primary interest is in the protection of minority privilege.

The chapter has also briefly discussed the emotional aspect of social movement formation. The authors mentioned above were interested in the power of emotion to the creation of a strong social dynamic. A more recent trend has been to focus on the negative power of emotions, with emphasis placed on the hurt caused to individuals and groups who are not being accorded full recognition of their humanity. This requires a more detailed discussion and is the subject of the next chapter.

Notes

1 Although Tilly is extremely critical of Durkheim, there are many similarities between his use of repertoires and some Durkheimian concepts. See Crossley (2002a) for a discussion on this.
2 It is worth noting that it is also becoming increasingly difficult for those in work to go on strike due to legal and bureaucratic measures that must be satisfied if the strike is to be deemed legal.

2   Recognizing identity

In 2001, shortly after I had taken up my current position with Manchester Metropolitan University, a speaker addressed my department's staff group on the theme of community participation. He told us to prepare for five questions, with the only proviso being that we could not give the same answer more than once. Question number one followed: Who are you? Then number two: Who are you? Number three: Who are you? Number four: Who are you? And the final question: Who are you?

The purpose of such a task is to get people to think about and identify the different aspects of their lives that make them who they are and what shapes their perception of themselves and their relationships with others. So, while most people respond to question one with their name, they are then forced to look beyond themselves for the remaining questions, considering how and with whom they interact at the interpersonal, social and cultural level.

Common answers include wife/husband/partner; gay/lesbian/straight; father/mother/carer; black/white; working/middle class; professional/sporty/friendly, and so on. Such an exercise indicates how the complex nature of identity is portrayed today, and of the interacting and at times competing nature of different identities, either at the individual or group level. The point being emphasized is that identities are not fixed or stable, but on the contrary are fluid, constantly changing and being reassessed, with various aspects of our identity being at the fore depending on the situation that we find ourselves in; for example a professional at work, a parent or partner once we return home.

An identity therefore gives an individual's life meaning by framing it in a social and historical context. It provides a bridge between current consciousness and past experiences. In a physical sense we may bear little resemblance in appearance to how we did when we were a child or adolescent but we still feel that we are the same person, that there is a continuous line from the past to the present. Aspects of our identity may have changed but our core identity as the same entity is reinforced. Self-interpretation leads people to an understanding of their experiences and of how these relate to their wider environment of family, friends, colleagues and formal institutions.

These self-aspects can refer to such things as generalized psychological characteristics or traits, physical features, role(s), abilities, tastes, attitudes, behaviours and explicit group membership (Simon 2004). Such an integrative approach takes into account the way in which people seek meaning in order to give coherence to their experiences. It is important to note that such self-aspects can be adapted and changed depending on context and further experience. For example, an experience, such as intervening to stop a crime, may make someone who previously considered themselves shy or timid to rethink that aspect of their identity. In addition, modern medical and cosmetic techniques can allow us to change our physical appearance and how we view ourselves, as the rise in breast enlargement for women, and the opposite procedure of breast reduction for men illustrates. Similarly, group membership or affiliation is subject to change; disillusionment with the New Labour government that came into power in 1997 led many people to rescind their party membership and seek political affiliation elsewhere.

This apparent split between social and personal identity is, of course, a false one, as a cursory reading of Freud, Marx, Lacan or Bourdieu, to name but a few, will confirm. It is in this regard that Simon (2004) prefers the terms 'collective' and 'individual' identity. An individual identity is not a purely internal asocial one, while collective identity is derived from *membership* in a collective or group and not the identity of a group as an objective entity. In other words it is a social relationship between the individual and a body of others. Subjectivity, from this perspective, is *situated subjectivity*, where our sense of self, our understanding of moral and ethical good, of what is just, are not ahistorical, universal phenomena but instead are inseparable from specific socio-cultural conditions, social contracts and interaction.

Whether a particular aspect of identity is considered as individual or social can be dependent on the social and historical context; for example, whether you are Protestant or Catholic in Ireland, and to a lesser extent Scotland, takes on a more collective form than it would in present day England, where it is more likely to be viewed as an individual, apolitical identity. This also illustrates the importance of historicity as religious persecution has a long and bloody history in many countries. Simon (2004) gives the example of wearing spectacles, which most would assume was individual in nature, and gives the hypothetical example of where such wearers were chosen for special treatment, perhaps because they were considered dangerous, a situation which may lead to some form of collective emerging among them. Of course, the former has happened, the Pol Pot regime in Cambodia executed spectacle wearers as supposed intellectuals, although the latter did not follow; no mass movement of the short-sighted emerged. Identity formation is therefore historical and contingent. A variety of factors influence our identity, it is malleable and different aspects of it can be emphasized or hidden depending on context. Simon (2004) also gives the example of a German national, who may emphasize the national aspect of their identity if the discussion is on football, given their success in several World Cups, but who may downplay their nationality if the discussion changes to the Holocaust. Similarly, many will be familiar with downplaying some of their political or cultural views at family gatherings for the sake of domestic harmony.

For our purposes we are particularly interested in what aspects of identity are emphasized for political gain, in the pursuit of political goals, whether that is in challenging the status quo or in consolidating present political arrangements. There is a need to look at two inter-related issues. First, we look at the ways in which political grievances are articulated by a variety of social actors as they attempt to make sense of their experiences, and second, it is necessary to look at some of the theoretical developments around identity, in particular political identity, in order to provide an understanding of the intellectual climate in which current identity affiliation is expressed today. Subsequent chapters will then link this with wider social, political and intellectual currents.

Identity and equality

A sense of identity has often been linked to a sense of injustice. In social terms this has taken the form of collective awareness of group maltreatment and inequality. Women, black people, homosexuals and the working class formed groups in recognition that they were not treated on an equal basis within society. Group formation and solidarity allowed what could be perceived or justified by the powerful as natural or valid distinctions, to be challenged as inequitable, unjust and socially constructed.

It is necessary to clarify, at this point, just what we mean by equality. It does not mean uniformity, that everyone should be the same, since this would rob us of our uniqueness; men and women, or the variety of ethnic groups do not have to merge into an undifferentiated hybrid, it is sufficient that neither is advantaged over the other. Likewise, equality in health does not mean that we all should suffer the same pain or die at the same age. Spicker (2006) identifies five forms of equality: equality of persons; equality of rights; citizenship; access to the 'conditions of civilization'; and equality of welfare. The denial of aspects of these is often a catalyst for social protest.

General or human rights are those that apply to everyone (usually within the nation state), so that irrespective of such things as age, ethnicity, gender or sexuality, each citizen enjoys, in theory at least, similar rights. Particular rights are those that only apply to certain people, contractual and employment rights for example. While it is the former that are our main concern, it should be noted that social movements also campaign to address inequities in the latter, for instance in trying to get work-based pension schemes (discretionary and therefore a particular right) made available to other employees. Human rights, such as those in the US Declaration of Independence of 'life, liberty and the pursuit of happiness' can be said to apply to citizens of all countries. Of course, behind the rhetoric lies the realpolitik, so the principle can easily be jettisoned in places such as Guantanamo Bay. It is also worth pointing out that the term 'human rights' has been criticized for being a discursive charade used to justify western intervention in the rest of the world; from this perspective, 'humanitarian intervention' replaces colonial rule.

National identity has a significant bearing on how you are treated, with rights depending to a greater or lesser extent on whether or not you are accorded citizenship of the country in which you are residing. Immigration laws, by their nature, are designed to be unequal by denying entry, or if entry is allowed imposing restrictions on length of stay, ability to work, recourse to public funds, etc. It can also allow those deemed illegal immigrants to be detained and/or deported.

In terms of equality and general rights, a recent expression of its extension to hitherto unrecognized groups is in relation to gay marriage, or civil partnerships as they are officially known in the UK. The rights and public recognition afforded to heterosexual married couples did not, indeed could not as the law stood, apply to same-sex partners. Consequently, their relationships were not afforded the same rights as those given to heterosexual couples, a discrepancy in treatment with very real as well as symbolic consequences. First, it implies that same-sex relationships lie outside the 'norm' of hetero-sexual ones, that there is therefore something abnormal within the gay relationship. Second, there are very real material consequences, for example in relation to pension entitlement and inheritance tax if one partner dies. The issue of sexuality and civil partnerships will be discussed in more detail below. For now it is sufficient to highlight that what is being demanded is that their relationship, one aspect of their identity, is afforded public *recognition*.

Society and identity

In terms of political engagement there has been not only a shift to 'identity' in contemporary social thought, but also a related move to have the chosen identity formally recognized and validated (Taylor 1994; Fraser 1995). However, as the above questions illustrate, our identities today are not a given. Whereas in previous societies identity was largely fixed according to social class or status, today by contrast we are said to be able to choose our identity reflexively from various competing aspects of our lives (Giddens 1990).

How we identify ourselves and our perception of how others view us does not therefore take place in a vacuum, rather it is shaped by social, cultural and political influences. For example, prior to the industrial revolution nobody would have identified themselves as working class, and while there has always been homosexual activity, the construction of the 'homosexual' is a relatively recent develop-ment, and without changing and more liberal attitudes to homo-sexuality it is questionable whether as many people would identify themselves as gay or lesbian. Repressive legislation and hostile social attitudes can lead to people remaining silent for fear of retribution. More recently, in relation to mental health policy and practice, there has been a rise in the number of people who identify themselves as users or 'survivors' of mental health services (Campbell 1996). Again, this development has been influenced by changing social mores that are more tolerant of behaviour that was once dismissed as 'mad', and segregated from the rest of society in the asylums.

This is not to say that such groups are now free from discrimi-nation. Many people will remain silent about any mental health problems they may have for fear of incarceration, victimization or losing their jobs, and homosexuals can still be attacked purely because of their sexuality. Relatively speaking however, the social accept-ability of such issues, certainly in the UK, is greater than at any time in the past century, making it easier for people to speak openly about their experiences and desires. Although, as we will discuss in subsequent chapters, there is a growing tendency whereby people are now *required* to speak about their experiences within specific identity categories, and such an identity-focused subjectivity can be past as opposed to future oriented, and necessitate the presentation of the self as a vulnerable entity.

Social change is therefore a major component in how we view ourselves today. How this interacts with intellectual concerns is also important. The argument put forward here is that a dialectical relationship is at work, an analysis of which allows us to locate both the progressive and problematic elements of contemporary discourse as it moves towards an increasing number of competing identities.

Intellectual life in the closing decades of the twentieth century was marked by a sense that major social change was off the political agenda. According to Fukuyama (1992), we had reached 'the end of history'. For him, the collapse of communism in Eastern Europe, most notably symbolized by the tearing down of the Berlin Wall, meant that the battle over how best to organize society had been won, with western liberal democracy proclaimed the victor. The vanquished included not only those social systems recently overthrown, but also by implication those in the west who espoused Marxist or socialist ideals. The historical struggle of ideas was over according to this reading. Of course, the decline in the revolutionary project in the West predated the fall of the Soviet bloc. The post-1968 generation gradually lost belief in the potential of the working class as the historic agent of history and began to look to other social movements to take forward the 'progressive project'; the class focus gradually receded with issues of culture around gender, sexuality and race gaining in priority. In this respect, the fall of the Berlin Wall in 1989 merely symbolized the end of a radical project that had been defeated many years previously.

The belief by some that we had reached an ideological impasse is in itself nothing new. Jacoby (1999) details this ideological decline and believes it is more stark today, but he also points out that such sentiments have a long pedigree, titling one chapter of his book 'The End of the End of the End of Ideology' to illustrate this point. However, the present time is marked not only by intellectual pessimism and a lack of ideological vision within the political elites but also by the demise of the working class as a political force. Crushing defeats in the 1980s, most notably the defeat of the miners' strike of 1984–85, falling union membership, fewer days lost to strikes, stand in contrast to the 1970s when unions were capable of bringing down governments (Upham 1996; Heartfield 2002). Although some see grounds for optimism in the 'anti-capitalist' or 'anti-globalization' movements, or indeed the celebration of 'identity', it is clear that the present epoch is markedly different from the preceding one.

If social change in the wider sense is no longer perceived as possible, then it follows that engagement and intervention can also only be of a limited nature. This note of pessimism also affects commentators such as Francis Fukuyama, whose 1992 book *The End of History* lacks the triumphalist tone of his article 'The End of History?' published in *The National Interest* journal only three years earlier. Fukuyama recognized that social problems can be modified at a micro level only if the macro system is beyond dispute. However, the decline in class politics and the ideologies that gave them coherence does not mean that the problems they attempted to address have been resolved. The political conflicts and tensions within contemporary society as experienced by the marginalized have not disappeared; they have merely taken on a different form. As others have noted (e.g. Taylor 1994; Fraser 1995), group identity and the politics of recognition are increasingly the medium through which these contradictions are channelled, with social injustice seen as one of cultural domination rather than of economic exploitation. It therefore follows that cultural recognition is seen as the main remedy for such injustice and becomes the focus of political struggle.

Fraser (1995) notes how the shift to 'identity', 'difference', 'cultural domination' and 'recognition' can be regarded as 'false consciousness', or as an attempt to redress the 'culture blindness' approach of more materialist paradigms. 'False consciousness' is a phrase usually used by socialists or Marxists to explain how the oppressed fail to see the source of their oppression as being due to the capitalist system, although the term can also expose a form of intellectual snobbery, as the 'enlightened' politicos see themselves as necessary to educate and lead the 'unenlightened' masses. The focus on economics and class was challenged by many for failing to adequately acknowledge the different forms that oppression could take, for example due to race, culture, sexuality and disability. From such a perspective, ignoring these differences is held to be a form of 'culture blindness'.

The move to a cultural form of politics based on the recognition of group specificity led at times to an antagonistic polarization between the 'new' recognition theorists and the 'old' economic redistributionists, each maintaining that their position required priority focus. Believing both approaches to be simplistic if seen in such isolationist terms, Fraser (1995) argues that redistribution and recognition are not mutually exclusive alternatives. For her, what is needed is 'a *critical theory* of recognition, one which identifies and defends only those versions of the cultural politics of difference that can be coherently combined with the social politics of equality' (Fraser 1995: 69, emphasis in original). Social justice for Fraser, then, needs not only cultural or group recognition but also economic and material redistribution. Economic injustice *and* cultural injustice need to be addressed.

What is 'cultural injustice'? For Fraser it includes

> cultural domination (being subjected to patterns of interpretation and communication that are associated with another culture and are alien and/or hostile to one's own); nonrecognition (being rendered invisible via the authoritative representational, communicative, and interpretive practices of one's culture); and disrespect (being routinely maligned or disparaged in stereotypic public cultural representations and/or in everyday interactions).
>
> (Fraser 1995: 71)

The demand for recognition is perhaps the most common form of redress in relation to these interrelated terms, with various cultural groups demanding that their specific values, beliefs, histories and practices be accorded social recognition. Examples of these would be lesbian and gay groups, black groups, disability groups and women's groups who challenged dominant representations of the 'normal' as being white, heterosexual, able-bodied and masculine. For them, their experiences, histories and narratives had been ignored, distorted and devalued by such normative representations, and therefore raising their voices would allow different and contested stories to emerge that would challenge the cultural and political orthodoxies of the day. The demand for recognition is here portrayed as giving a voice to those hitherto silenced by the powerful; their experiences, differences and histories are now to be 'recognized' as valid.

In and of itself, this desire for recognition is not a new theoretical or intellectual insight, although its articulation has changed from one of struggle to a more therapeutically oriented demand for recognition. Hegel identified the struggle for recognition as the primary motor of human history some two hundred years ago, arguing that it was not an economic struggle, but a desire to be recognized that propelled people to try to surpass their circumstances and be recognized by others. It is necessary not only for the individual to recognize others but also for them in turn to be recognized by others. Such a reciprocal relationship of mutual recognition is therefore held to be necessary in obtaining full human subjectivity. Fukuyama (1992: 144) draws on Hegelian theory to argue that while economic accounts of history have their place, the 'recognition' thesis provides a 'totally non-materialist historical dialectic that is much richer in its understanding of human motivation' than any Marxist economic or sociological explanations for human action. Fukuyama, a champion of western liberal democracy, sees capitalist competition as the contemporary arena for the desire for recognition to take place, with material and economic success, academic status, peer or social approval being primarily led by a desire to be recognized as worthwhile, as a success.

Hegel has also been read as implying that an equal society is necessary for worthwhile recognition to flourish. The weak may be unrecognized, but the powerful, who gain their recognition from the weak, realize that such recognition from the unrecognized is worthless. Hegel's master–slave dialectic then can be read for the contemporary age as the struggle between winner and loser:

> Those who fail to win out in the honor stakes remain unrecognized. But even those who do win are more subtly frustrated, because they win recognition from the losers, whose acknowledgement is, by hypothesis, not really valuable, since they are no longer free, self supporting subjects on the same level with the winners. The struggle for recognition can find only one satisfactory solution, and that is a regime of reciprocal recognition among equals.
>
> (Taylor 1994: 50)

In Fraser's view, Hegel is instructive in what his thesis tells us about those who are not afforded recognition or who are subject to misrecognition. She sees the essence of misrecognition as 'the material construction through the institutionalization of cultural norms of a class of devalued persons who are impeded from participatory parity' (Fraser 2008: 62). Such misrecognition has been the fate of many marginal groups and in this respect the demand for recognition involves a struggle for *social* justice alongside equitable economic distribution. If the current discussion over identity takes the form of recognition of one's vulnerability, this is, for some, the very essence of Hegel's dialectic. For Butler (2004), the life and death struggle for recognition, described by Hegel in 'Lordship and Bondage' as being when two self-consciousnesses come to recognize the other and also that they have the power to obliterate the other, paradoxically also destroys the condition of their own self-reflection, and with it their own self. From this perspective, the very moment of recognition is one of 'fundamental vulnerability'. This notion of 'fundamental vulnerability' will be pursued in Chapter 3 in relation to the therapeutic turn in political life and identity formation.

That recognition is the primary condition for a meaningful life does not mean that lack of recognition is necessarily negative. It can, on the contrary, lead to a struggle for recognition that aims to overcome the destruction of negation by way of individual or collective attempts to achieve such recognition. Honneth (2003), one of the main proponents of the recognition thesis, argues that the desire for recognition is akin to a primal need, a universal constant throughout history, one that is so fundamental to individual self-realization that its pursuit is the primary motivating force behind social development. Misrecognition then can lead to a struggle for recognition (Fraser and Honneth 2003). For example, Butler is fully aware of how aspects of her identity as a woman and lesbian are not accorded recognition, or to be more accurate are accorded deviant status. She found herself, like many minority or oppressed people, being seen as 'Other', and felt herself to occupy the term she was interrogating (Butler 2004: 240). Such negation of her humanity, while destructive, also leads her to use such negation in pursuit of change, a change that is necessary not purely on the basis of human dignity but of life itself. As she puts it, 'gaining recognition for one's status as a sexual minority is a difficult task within reigning discourses of law, politics and language, I continue to consider it a necessity for survival' (Butler 2004: xxvi).

The aforementioned campaigns for civil partnerships were concerned with having an important part of one's identity recognized as being worthy of public celebration and affirmation. Analysing the results of various responses to the proposals for civil partnerships, Spicker (2006) found opinions varied, from those who saw it as a simple matter of equality, extending the rights enjoyed by heterosexuals to homosexuals (which would also reduce stigma and homophobia), to those who were unhappy because it did not go far enough (civil partnership falling short of marriage). Opposition mainly, but not exclusively, came from the conservative and religious right who condemn all moves to accord homosexuality any form of legitimacy or recognition. However, within the lesbian and gay movement there were also tensions over the pros and cons of elevating marriage within same-sex relationships as the desired norm, as the standard required for public legitimation.

Confronting the homophobic arguments by arguing for those in same-sex relationships to be granted the same rights to marry as heterosexuals can inadvertently re-establish marriage as the norm, as something to which all committed long-term relationships ought to aspire. This dilemma has exercised Butler, who notes how it reinforces marriage, family and kinship relations as the exclusive terrain on which sexual relations are discussed and legitimized; the field of sexuality still 'being gauged against the marriage norm' (Butler 2004: 130). As one form of sexual relationship is allowed into the fold of 'correct sexual relations', it has the effect of further marginalizing those sexual relationships that do not wish to be defined in such a way. Defining kinship ties as heterosexual, or both hetero and homosexual, is also, according to Butler, to ignore the many kinship ties that are not about enduring or exclusive sexual relations – community or kinship ties can include ex-lovers, non-lovers, friends and community members.

Today's demands, then, are concerned with more than gaining some 'respect' out of common courtesy. There is a belief that the negative stereotypes portrayed are harmful to the self worth of the individual or group who can internalize such sentiments. Taylor (1994) notes how this perspective views lack of recognition, or *misrecognition*, as being more than a failure to show respect, rather, misrecognition can 'inflict a grievous wound, saddling its victims with a crippling self hatred. . . . Due recognition therefore is not just a courtesy we owe people. It is a vital human need' (Taylor 1994: 26). Such analyses draw not only on the therapeutic notion of 'self-esteem' but also on Foucauldian ideas of how discourse represents and maintains existing power relations. For the oppressed, or in this case the 'misrecognized', 'their own self-deprecation becomes one of the most potent instruments of their own oppression' (Taylor 1994: 26). If the desire for recognition is what makes us human, it follows that not being recognized will have a detrimental effect on our self-image. This is the idea discussed by Taylor who argues that recognition is necessary for the concept of a healthy self-identity. In this interpretation, the withholding of recognition is harmful to the individual or group's self-image; internalizing hostile attitudes as a consequence of non-recognition leads to low self esteem and a damaged identity. The withholding of recognition in this way by state authorities, or experiencing hostility by individuals due to this, is therefore seen to be a form of oppression. From such a perspective political prioritization is given to the pursuit of recognition.

Redistribution or recognition?

The apparent dichotomy between a political approach focused on redistributive politics and one that emphasizes the need for cultural recognition is one that has taxed many political theorists and activists, particularly in this 'post-socialist age' (Fraser 1995). Fraser's work has developed in response to many critiques and debates (e.g. Fraser and Honneth 2003; Fraser 2008). Her primary concern is that according primacy to struggles over recognition risks downplaying at best, dismissing at worst, the struggle for economic redistribution that has been the normative mode of theoretical thought and effort since Marx.

Indeed, in terms of material wealth, the world is a vastly unequal place, and despite unprecedented total wealth the distribution of it has certainly not been equal. For example, from 1960 to 1997 the ratio of the wealthiest 20 per cent of the world's population compared to the poorest 20 per cent had risen from 60:1 to 74:1 (UNDP 1999). Of course the poorest 20 per cent may have more material benefits than in the past, so in absolute terms they are wealthier than they were previously, but in terms of relative wealth their status has decreased. Inequality with regards to economic distribution is still a cause for concern, so Fraser is right to be wary of marginalizing it as an issue.

It is not that recognition theorists are unaware of this as a potential problem. Honneth himself argues that any critical theory concerned with being 'able to understand itself as a theoretical reflection of the emancipatory movements of the age . . . should develop a normative frame of reference in which the two competing objectives of recognition and redistribution both receive their due' (Honneth 2003: 112). Nevertheless, whereas Fraser sees a synthesis between both positions as being the normative objective of critical social theory, for Honneth the terms of recognition must present the unified framework for such a project. In essence, Honneth subsumes redistribution into the recognition paradigm because he sees material social inequality as a distributional injustice, as the 'institutional expression of social disrespect –, or better said, of unjustified relations of recognition' (Honneth 2003: 114).

In doing so, however, Honneth prioritizes the psychological over the material and in a sense contributes to the therapeutic turn in contemporary political life. He accurately notes the danger within the normative political tradition, whereby only those aspects of human suffering that have been politicized/publicized by media-savvy organizations are recognized as legitimate concerns. This can ignore those socially unjust beliefs and practices that have, thus far, been deprived of public recognition. Indeed, many new social movements, most notably feminism, worked to bring to public attention the hitherto unrecognized ways in which their experiences were demeaned and marginalized and their bodies objectified. It is certainly the case that as one political movement or issue gains prominence, by implication other concerns are relatively downgraded in the public political sphere. However, Honneth's concern for unrecognized, unarticulated hurt risks individualizing the political sphere and missing what is specific about contemporary society that has influenced such articulation, namely that articulating misrecognition is not only a psychological and political process, but also a historical and material one.

By contending that the desire for recognition is both timeless and universal, Honneth lacks historical grounding and his telos of self-realization is also open to question. For example, Christopher Zurn asks why self-realization is necessarily the principal ideal of social organization: 'Why self-realization and not pious self-abnegation, or virtuous subservience to communal ends, or righteous obedience to the moral law, or maximization of the pleasure of others, etc?' (quoted in McNay 2008: 133). In addition, a Foucauldian perspective would see the contemporary desire for recognition as a form of governmentality, a form of control that harbours certain ways of relating to both ourselves and others. Therefore,

> what Honneth regards as the spontaneous and innate nature of the desire for recognition is an example of how, in late modernity, disciplinary structures have been so thoroughly internalized by individuals, that they have become self-policing subjects. In similar fashion, Bourdieu understands recognition as an internalized misrecognition of the inequalities of social existence.
>
> (McNay 2008: 133)

In drawing our attention to the need for an integrated approach, Fraser (2003) points out how 'class' is conceptualized as a mode of social stratification rooted in the political-economic structure. Fraser does not conceive of class in conventional Marxist terms of a relation to the means of production, but as one of economic inequality whereby some actors are denied the means and resources necessary for *participatory parity*. To rectify this, a policy of redistribution, not recognition, is necessary. In fact, following Marxist theory through, the object of the exercise is to abolish class society and hence working class identity; recognition of class specificity is not the goal of emancipatory class politics. Fraser also acknowledges that while class injustice is rooted in the economic sphere, it can also encompass elements of status injury as the working class are demeaned in a materialist oriented society.

The other extreme is that of a collectivity solely rooted in culture, where the root of the injustice suffered by the group is one of cultural misrecognition, or status injury. While doubting the existence of any such culturally exclusive collectivity, Fraser, for heuristic purposes, considers homosexuality. As homosexuals occupy all spheres of social differentiation in class society then their mode of collectivity is based not on their relationship to the means of production, but rather on their position as a devalued group. Their marginalization due to heterosexist societal norms, of being subject to harassment, violence and discrimination is therefore, according to Fraser, one of cultural devaluation. While she acknowledges that homosexuals can also suffer serious economic injustices, for example being refused employment due to their sexuality,[1] and being denied heteronormative family-based social-welfare benefits, these are seen not as being rooted directly in the economic structure, but as deriving from an unjust cultural-valuational structure.

This contention that homosexuality is devalued primarily due to cultural misrecognition is disputed by some, who take exception to the depiction of issues around sexuality as being 'merely cultural'. Butler (2008) argues that Fraser's downgrading of queer politics in this way derives from an analysis that overlooks the way in which, in a capitalist economy, the regulation of sexuality, with all its gendered heterosexist assumptions was systematically tied to the mode of economic production. In this way, both 'gender' and 'sexuality' become part of material life, 'not only because of the way in which it serves the sexual division of labor, but also because normative gender serves the reproduction of the normative family' (Butler 2008: 51). Drawing on Althusser's argument that 'an ideology always exists in an apparatus, and its practice, or practices. This existence is material' (Althusser 1971: 166), Butler concludes that 'even if homophobia were conceived only as a cultural attitude, that attitude should still be located in the apparatus and practice of its institutionalization' (Butler 2008: 54). Indeed, she goes further in that for her, the question is not one of whether sexual politics belong to the economic or cultural sphere, but that it destabilizes the distinction between both spheres.

The consequences of both these extremes of redistribution and recognition require different remedies. In the former, the aim is to put the collective out of business, to eradicate the working class as a specific group by abolishing the class system. With the latter, however, the aim is to recognize the group's specificity. Things become more complicated when we consider cases where bivalent collectivities are considered, in which an identity combines economic exploitation with degraded cultural valuation. Fraser specifically discusses gender and race in relation to this bivalency. Women suffer economic exploitation due to the differentiation of labour, with women traditionally occupying the lower or unpaid employment sphere. They can also suffer due to cultural problems around objectification, sexual exploitation, violence and harassment. Similarly, race also combines both, being a structural principle of political and economic development, more so in the past but still with relevance today, and also of cultural devaluation due to racism and eurocentrism.

The question of what is truly political and what is 'merely cultural' is not a new one for feminism. Marxist arguments were similarly criticized for viewing gender, and indeed other forms of oppression, as being of less importance than economic class focused ones, the former seen as more related to the realm of culture. In his contribution to the debate, Rorty (2008) notes how the central left idea that we all share a common humanity did not pay much consideration to the notion that marginalized groups such as black people, women and manual workers possessed a distinct culture,[2] apart from those Marxists who almost celebrated 'working class' culture. Overall, Rorty (2008) approves of the term 'recognition' as encapsulating what we all need from each other – to be recognized as full human beings regardless of our race, class, gender, sexual orientation or other social difference. As such 'the need for recognition' can combine various new social movements in a more apposite way than 'the need to eliminate prejudice' allows. However, he is less clear about, and not entirely supportive of, the way the term 'recognition' has come 'to be thought of as recognition of *culture* or of "cultural differences", rather than as recognition of a common humanity' (Rorty 2008: 71, emphasis in original).

In attempting to account for this move from recognition of a common humanity to recognition of cultural difference, Rorty (2008) implicates the academic Left and the retreat to the academy. The defeat of the Left in the latter decades of the twentieth century, and intellectual disillusionment with the working class as it failed to fulfil its historical role as the agent of revolutionary change, led some to pursue the radical agenda through the academy rather than society, and to look to other groups in order to carry the radical banner forward. However, although an academic's ability to instigate meaningful social change is limited, by writing about and celebrating certain cultural groups' histories and practices he or she could make some attempt to remove prejudice. Rorty certainly has a point, and much progress was made in changing attitudes towards hitherto devalued groups, although the role of academic activists should not be overstated. The new social movements had more than a little to do with instigating such change themselves, helped in part by a loss of confidence by the establishment in upholding its more 'traditional' values. However, given the collapse of class politics and the ideologies that gave them coherence, the liberal elite arguably have a greater influence today than previously in driving the political/cultural agenda, as they to a great extent fill the ideological and political vacuum left by the loss of previous political outlooks.

What Rorty (2008) is trying to do is work out how to get to a situation where people and children are taught that, for example, to be gay or straight, black or white is no big deal, rather than to accord 'positive recognition' to devalued groups, or of it being obligatory to learn about the merits of any particular culture. Others are also acutely aware that such affirmation of group specificity risks not only reifying identities, but also of the apparent paradox that,

> The socioeconomic injustices associated with gender and race are best remedied by putting race and gender out of business as categories: restructuring the division of labor and income so that people's position in social and economic relations is no longer dictated by their gender or race. But the cultural injustices – 'the pervasive devaluation of things coded as "feminine", and of things coded as "black", "brown"', and "yellow"' – seem to require a positive revaluation of the characteristics of the despised groups, a stronger affirmation of their group identity.
>
> (Philips 2008: 119)

This concern with the problem of reification and tendency towards the essentialism of identity has been discussed by many other writers. Taylor, for example, has been criticized for viewing identities as integral and authentic which can overlook the complex internal and external social and psychological dynamics through which identities are formed. The attempt to grasp such complexities through a single framework of 'cultural recognition' can also conflate individual and community unity, when these can be, and often are, in conflict (Wolf 1994). It can also homogenize communities, for example in the way 'community leaders' purport to speak on behalf of 'their' community as if there is no difference in beliefs, values and political outlook within such communities. In addition, the false unity imputed to diverse struggles can also lead to a normalizing and conservative outlook in which the past, by way of tradition, is used to discipline the behaviour of subjects in the present by enforcing moral codes of behaviour that uphold the status quo and problematic social relations. This danger was noted by Appiah (1994) when he pointed out that there is no clear demarcation between a politics based on recognition and one based on compulsion. In other words, it is but a short step from cultural tradition favouring an individual behaving in a certain way to insisting that the individual behave in the 'traditional' way.

From insult to injury

In attempting to overcome the problem of reification and relativism within identity/recognition politics, whereby any group can claim a historical or cultural right to demand affirmative recognition in the case of many, or to be left alone free from state intrusion in the case of some, Fraser argues that we need to reinterpret recognition in terms of *status*. Consequently she argues that we need to view misrecognition as *status injury* or *status subordination* rather than the psychological injury approach favoured by Honneth. From this perspective,

> what requires recognition is not group-specific identity but rather the status of individual group members as full partners in social interaction. Misrecognition, accordingly, does not mean the depreciation of group identity. Rather, it means *social subordination* in the sense of being prevented from participating as a peer in social life as a result of institutionalized patterns of cultural value that constitute one as relatively unworthy of respect or esteem. To redress the injustice requires a politics of recognition, but this does not mean identity politics. On the status model, rather, it means a politics aimed at overcoming subordination by *deinstitutionalizing patterns of cultural value that impede parity of participation and replacing them with patterns that foster it.*
>
> (Fraser 2008: 84, emphasis in original)

Culture, in this reading, is only an object of political concern when institutionalized forms of cultural valuation deny some social actors the right to participate fully and equally in social life. Affirming the distinctiveness of a specific cultural group would be judged to the degree or otherwise that it extends participatory parity.

The danger of essentializing identity is acknowledged by writers such as Taylor. Indeed, his dialogical account of identity formation is an attempt to avoid the dangers of such a pitfall. However, it is not so much the essentialist nature of Taylor's work that is the main problem, but his failure to capture the way in which power and identity formation are coexistent rather than sequential. As McNay points out, such an error means his

> linguistic version of the recognition model of subject formation is divorced from an account of power. On his view, power relations are secondary to the formation of identity in language, instead of being regarded as coeval with it. This detachment of language from power allows Taylor to isolate the expressive function of language as its primal *modus operandi* and, as a consequence, to foreclose an analysis of how self-expression is constitutively shaped by power relations.
>
> (McNay 2008: 69)

The same criticism is levelled at Habermas, whom McNay accuses of failing to adequately recognize that the subject's entry into language coexists with entry into existing power relations. Whereas for Bourdieu, language and power are inseparable, Habermas's assertion that the telos of language is an orientation to understanding implies that power is extrinsic to language. Language and power are not sequential, one does not follow the other, rather they are coeval. In order to overcome this problem McNay draws on the work of Bourdieu, and in particular his notion of *habitus*

> as a way of explaining how power relations are incorporated into the body as physical and psychological dispositions, habitus prevents the naturalization of the cluster of emotions associated with social suffering that is the consequence of Honneth's ontology of recognition.
>
> (McNay 2008: 127)

This notion of embodied subjectivity is similar to the dialogical conception proposed by thinkers of recognition, but is located more within a sociological account of power that allows us to gain a better grasp of subject formation than could otherwise be obtained. It is not that Bourdieu is indifferent to the powerful effect language can have on subject formation, on the contrary he views it as extremely important, but he locates language itself as formed through powerful social dynamics. In other words, he sees it as embodied in a social context. Likewise, Habermas is not unaware of the distorting effects of power on language and therefore on the possibility of achieving an 'ideal speech' situation. He outlines a variety of conditions to allow equal communicative participation. It is more that his strategic solutions are ineffectual because he views power as a post hoc distortion of pure understanding. If the Habermasian telos is an orientation towards understanding then power must be extrinsic to language, whereas for Bourdieu, power is seen as 'ineluctably inscribed upon bodies and embedded in the structure of speech' (McNay 2008: 85–86). Without an adequate understanding of the way power relations are embodied and somatized, it is all too easy to miss the way in which 'the neutral language of rational discourse is in fact the *imposed* discourse of the cultural elite which has been naturalized through processes of inculcation' (McNay 2008: 86, my emphasis). An example of an identity being imposed from above is specifically discussed in Chapter 6 in relation to the legal construction of the 'vulnerable adult'.

In this respect, the subjectivism of Honneth's recognition thesis overlooks the diversity and historical specificity of political conflicts by 'falsely unifying them as manifestations of a basic ontological struggle', and by the setting up of an analytic dichotomy between culture and economy that 'disconnects identities from their material conditions' (McNay 2008: 161). Fraser's analysis overcomes these difficulties but at the cost of a satisfactory analysis of social agency, of what makes social actors coalesce around certain demands rather than others. This is due to her analysis focusing on those already existing socio-political movements with relatively little regard for their conditions of emergence.

Conclusion

The question that remains to be answered is why expressive recognition, or a more therapeutically centred view of subjectivity has come to the fore today. It could be that the recognition theorists provide a more optimistic account of subjectivity, one where mutual recognition can be obtained, as opposed to poststructuralist theorists' rejection of any possibility of subject unity, far less subject–object unification. The former tend towards inclusivity, the latter towards exclusivity. As McNay notes:

> Poststructuralism views subject formation as taking place through the exclusionary dynamic of the constitutive other. The 'illusion' of stable subjectivity is maintained only through a derogation or denial of the potentially troubling alterity of the other. Theories

of recognition tend to stress conversely the inclusive features of subject formation, that is, stable subjectivity is based on the ability to tolerate and embrace the other's difference. A significant implication of the inclusionary recasting of dialogical subjectivity is that it seemingly institutes an inalienable ethical bond to the other at the heart of normative thought.

(McNay 2008: 4)

It is in this regard, notwithstanding the valuable contributions of such theorists, that there is a need to consider what has allowed certain articulations of hurt to be accorded higher cultural recognition today than in the past, and more specifically for our purposes, there is the additional question of what factors lie behind individual and group demands to be recognized as a 'survivor'. The demand for recognition has become a defining paradigm of individual and political struggle today, but in a peculiar way, as a therapeutic mode of understanding whereby problems in living are viewed through a psychological prism, and where increasing numbers of people seek public affirmation of their suffering. Such a move cannot be fully explained at the level of theoretical abstraction discussed above, no matter how insightful such contributions are. Theoretical developments alone cannot adequately account for the rise of the politics of recognition; an account of social and political change is also necessary, as is an understanding of their interpenetration. So, while McNay's Bourdieu-inspired analysis of power, habitus and embodied subjectivity improves our understanding of the recognition debate, it pays insufficient attention to current articulations of identity and recognition in relation to recent social and political changes.

In this respect, there is a need for greater historical specificity to situate the discussion in a more concrete way. In the following chapters I wish to look at some societal developments and at how they have shaped our perceptions of both individual and social problems. As discussed earlier, of significance is the evacuation of the masses, in particular the working class from the political stage; their place taken by a new middle class, including academics and professionals, who now dominate public discourse and who, despite their claims to speak on behalf of the oppressed, constitute a new cultural elite. In addition, the primacy accorded specific identities today can lead to a focus on the past as opposed to the present, which is contrary to the intention of many of the initial proponents of identity politics. For them, identity was a project, a means to an end, not an inheritance from the past to be kept intact in the present and resistant to future change.

In order to illuminate these developments, the next chapter takes a more specific look at those social movements whose members identify as survivors. The aim is to ascertain the influence of the wider social dynamic on their formation, and to provide an understanding of how they perceive their problems and the strategies for self and/or social change that follow from such a conceptualization. As will be shown, a therapeutic form of recognition and the acknowledgement of hurt and trauma developed from the extremes of human behaviour, most specifically the Jewish experience of the Holocaust, to become the paradigm for the expression of contemporary political demands around both personal and political recognition.

Notes

1 While anti-discrimination legislation would prevent this from being given as the official reason today, certainly in the UK, it would be naive to think that certain employers would not hide such a decision under another guise.
2 It is worth noting that the notion that each group possesses a 'distinct culture' also risks essentializing such groups and minimising the complex differences within and between them.

3   Surviving trauma

Writing in 1984, Lasch identified the tendency towards a 'survival mentality' in western society whereby 'everyday life has begun to pattern itself on the survival strategies forced on those exposed to extreme adversity' and he noted how we were witnessing 'the normalization of crisis' (Lasch 1984: 57, 60), with almost every issue being presented as one of life-threatening potential, and of how such things as guidebooks, consumer products and media outlets increasingly promoted their wares on the basis that they could help you 'survive' some perceived hazard or life situation. This preoccupation crossed the political divide. For example, a left-wing magazine in the USA advertised itself as a 'survival guide' to the political years of the Ronald Reagan administration, while an anti-feminist group published a tract titled *A Survival Guide for the Bedeviled Male*. This trend continued to such an extent that thirty years later there were over one thousand self-help books with the word 'surviving' in the title, focusing, as Lasch no doubt would have expected, not on the extremes of human experience but on the more mundane, if unpleasant, aspects of life. Citing such titles as *Crazy Time: Surviving Divorce and Building a New Life*, *Surviving an Affair*, *The Girl's Guide to Surviving a Break Up* and *Surviving Motherhood*, Furedi (2004: 29) points out that 'coping with relatively banal, unexceptional episodes is now represented as an act of survival'. As was noted in the Introduction, such is the ubiquity of the term that even books that are critical of the medicalization of human experience and therapeutic culture can inadvertently tap into the survivalist consciousness, Smail's (1996) book being titled *How to Survive without Psychotherapy*.

This chapter looks the rise of the 'survivor' in relation to its usage initially to describe those who had endured the most horrendous experiences, to its adoption by a variety of groups to achieve either personal change, group solidarity or political goals, or a combination of all three, with each expressing a similar desire for wider public recognition.

The rise of the survivor

According to DeGloma, 'the very term "survivor" directly implies a history that includes child sex abuse, rape, the Holocaust or another atrocity' (DeGloma undated: 19). This may have been the case initially but many of today's 'survivors' need not have experienced such horrors. The prerequisite for becoming a survivor has changed from the endurance of extreme experiences to a rather more elastic one of suffering past or present victimization and/or form of personal distress.

In recent years, many experiences, while no doubt distressful to the individual concerned, but which bear no comparison to those cited by DeGloma, are now held to be ones which have been 'survived'. As the subject of past abuse began to be something that could be spoken about more openly within society, further accounts were heard from people who also declared themselves to be survivors. For example, there followed accounts from male victims of sexual abuse and the 'male survivor' (Mendel 1995). There is a growing movement of 'psychiatric survivors' (Campbell 1996). Indeed, the survivor suffix is used promiscuously today. Asylum seekers and refugees are held to be 'trauma survivors' (Weaver and Burns 2001), the testimonies of 'prostitution survivors' have been detailed (Sanders 2009), there are 'homelessness survivors' (Brandon et al. 1980), old-age survivors (Melucci 1992), cult survivors (Durocher 1999) and forced marriage survivors (Chantler et al. 2009) among others.

According to one account a survivor can be 'a person with a current or past experience of psychiatric hospital, recipients of ECT, tranquillizers, and other medication, users of counselling and therapy services' (quoted in Sayce 2000: 9). Although Sayce is primarily concerned with psychiatric survivors, given the extension of the trauma paradigm and the proliferation of therapy and counselling into more and more areas of daily life, it would appear that almost anyone can be defined, or more importantly, can define themselves, as a 'survivor'.

Exodus International is an organization that promotes 'freedom from homosexuality through the power of Jesus Christ'. Prayer will 'cure' the homosexual and make him/her an 'ex-gay'.[1] Several who have been through Exodus International's programme, and who found it not quite so easy to repress their desires for people of the same sex, have set up an 'Ex-gay survivor' group, holding conferences and workshops condemning Exodus's ministries as being emotionally and spiritually damaging (Roberts 2007). There are now 'verbal abuse survivors' groups, whose members can have survived 'disparaging remarks about one's gender' (quoted in Haaken 1998: 127). Name calling, according to Evans (1993), is abusive because it objectifies the recipient, and she has written books and set up a website to raise awareness of the 'problem' of verbal abuse. Evans claims that 'batterers define their mates as objects. It isn't healthy to be in the same room with a person who defines you, and it is harmful to children who witness it' (Evans undated). By using the term 'batterers' and emphasizing the harmful effects on children of witnessing such abuse, Evans seeks not only to emphasize the seriousness of the problem by linking verbal with physical abuse, but also to invoke fears over child safety to emphasize the need to seek escape and professional support.

There are also what could be termed *vicarious survivors*, those who were not directly affected by the traumatic experience but who have nevertheless suffered. This is most clearly illustrated in the growing numbers of second, and even third generation, Holocaust survivors. Such individuals and groups claim that they have suffered as a result of the trauma suffered by their parents or grandparents. This trans-generational trauma is held to have been detrimental to their own development. Similarly, parents of sexually abused children have formed support groups to help them deal with their own feelings because, 'We are all survivors like our children' (Baghramian and Kershaw 1989: 20).

In addition, there are many groupings today that gain great media coverage in their efforts to influence the political or judicial process. These groups often emerge out of tragic incidents, whether by acts of terrorism, accident or malpractice. Often it is the survivors themselves who form a collective. At other times, following fatal tragedies, it is the surviving relatives who come together to fight on behalf of their deceased loved ones. Examples of this would include the relatives of those Liverpool football fans who died at Hillsborough in 1989; the relatives of the victims of the Pan Am flight that blew up over Lockerbie in 1988; the injured victims and relatives of those who died in the London suicide bombings in 2005; the relatives and supporters of the Bloody Sunday shootings in Derry, Northern Ireland in 1972. With the exception of the last event, whose members may have been already active in Irish republican or civil rights activism, such group-ings are not so much social movements as *arbitrary aggregates*. Their existence is not the result of the consciousness of societal oppression due to an ascribed identity, but is because they or their relatives were in the wrong place at the wrong time. They do not share a common history but a direct experience; they have, sometimes literally, been thrown together. For these groupings, the term 'survivor' also serves to endow the speaker with moral authority; as a victim who has survived, their view is meant to be taken seriously.

It can be seen that there has been a growth in the survivor suffix in relation to the number of individual and group survivors, and also the variety and extent of experiences that are seen as something that has been survived. In similar vein, the experience of the Holocaust has almost become the prism through which much of human adversity is viewed today. The primary focus on it as a tragedy for the Jewish community is challenged by other groups who wish to highlight that their specific group identity also suffered in the Nazi concentration camps. Disability groups, homosexuals and gypsies, for example, have all demanded recognition for their plight during this period.

In addition, the term Holocaust does not now just refer to the one specific event of the Second World War but is now used more liberally to describe many more experiences. The horror of the Holocaust carries great emotional power and its usage 'has been co-opted and transferred to other experiences, such as the African-American Holocaust, the Serbian Holocaust, the Bosnian Holocaust or the Rwandan Holocaust' (Furedi 2004: 151). In similar vein, anti-abortion activists talk about a Holocaust of foetuses, while animal-rights activists highlight the Holocaust of animals. Some go so far as to link the Nazi Holocaust and ecological issues, arguing that we are witnessing an 'ecological Holocaust' the creation of 'planet Auschwitz'. In such a reading, the contemporary Hitler is someone who has 'so violated the bounds of humanity that they . . . are no longer my neighbour, or someone with whom I can identify, or anything but a rabid cancer on the body of the ecosystem'. The contemporary Hitler's crime: to 'continue to produce ozone-destroying CFCs' (Gottlieb 1994).

The term Holocaust is now frequently used in an attempt to give legitimacy to whatever moral or political view the protagonists adhere to. Even sociologists of the Holocaust can be apologetic for focusing on it. For example, while Gerson and Wolf (2007: 4) note that today the term survivor can pertain to almost anything 'from someone who was a victim of incest to someone who remains employed after a corporate merger', they themselves consider it problematic to use the phrase '*the* Holocaust, setting it up as the sole, most important holocaust and the standard for other holocausts' (Gerson and Wolf 1997: 9, emphasis in original). In line with postmodernist thinking, just as there is no 'Truth' (with a capital T) but myriad 'truths' (with a small t), there is no Holocaust, only myriad holocausts.

The proliferation of survivor organizations and individuals willing to identify with them is relatively unquestioned. For example, in otherwise informative contributions on mental health issues, commentators rarely question the concept of surviving, or when they do it is in relation to it in literal terms, pointing out that there are many people who will not 'survive', either by way of suicide or long term confinement in hospital or community home (Sayce 2000). The term user/survivor can be detached from any discussion as to its wider cultural roots in such a way that these developments are cast in a wholly positive light with the movements said to

> enable their members to speak as experts on their own lives, rather than remaining the 'objects' of the expert-knowledge claims of others. The discourses of survivors and users of the psychiatric system set up a *counter-discourse* to both psychology and industry.
> (Spandler and Batsleer 2000: 174, my emphasis)

Nevertheless, the 'survivor' discourse does not take place in a vacuum, but rather is shaped by wider influences. The proliferation of such groups indicates that there has been a cultural shift in how people relate to past and present distressful events. And while some commentators see their rise as a challenge to the dominant disciplines of psychiatry and psychology, to a remarkable extent such groups embrace psychological interpretations and interventions in their accounts of both the causes and 'cures' of human distress. The counter-discourse is more accurately described as a parallel discourse.

There has been an expansion of the 'psy-complex' in society, a development that has partly contributed to all manner of human interactions being reinterpreted as psychologically damaging and requiring therapeutic intervention to soothe the damaged psyche. The discourse of trauma and the testimonies of those who have survived it have gone mainstream. In order to understand this development it is necessary to look at the history of the 'survivor', one linked by the Holocaust and, to a significant degree, a therapeutically orientated form of feminism.

Holocaust survivors and the second generation

Initially, the term 'survivor' referred almost exclusively to those suffering trauma as a result of their experiences in the Nazi concentration camps. In this sense, its use as an identity label denotes past victimization, either as an individual or a group. It is, however, difficult to delineate the precise genealogy of the term. Its usage was rare until the 1960s (Cohen 2007). Many of those who had literally survived the camps and moved abroad tended to prefer the term immigrant over refugee or survivor, as this implied active agency rather than passive victimhood; the *immigrant* being someone who exhibited agency in choosing to migrate, whereas the use of the term refugee referred to constraints and expulsion (Gerson 2007). Nevertheless, it is possible to identify some key influences on the growth of the survivor suffix.

In *The Survivor: An Anatomy of Life in the Death Camps* about the testimonies of those who survived the Nazi Holocaust, Terrence Des Pres defines survival as 'the capacity of men and women to live beneath the pressure of protracted crisis, to sustain terrible damage in mind and body and yet be there, sane, alive, still human' (Des Pres 1980: v). What emerges from Holocaust survivor testimonies is their desire to survive not only in a literal sense but also in order to be a witness to the atrocities that were committed, to let the world know what had happened, to speak out on behalf of the dead. However, such testimonies were rarely heard in public forums in the immediate post-war years. With some exceptions, the direct Holocaust survivors mostly remained silent about their experiences, even to family and close friends. There was little private discourse around the Holocaust, far less the public one that is familiar to most of us today. The horrors of the Holocaust may not have been spoken aloud by the actual survivors, but for some of their children its impact was severe, as they were 'raised in a psychological atmosphere poisoned by the scarring that their survivor parents have brought to their child-rearing tasks' (Chodoff 1997: 155). Many of these children were of the belief that they themselves had been damaged as a result of their parents' Holocaust experience. One study in which 55 descendants of Holocaust survivors were interviewed found that they had a lack of knowledge about their parents' experiences, although the presence of the past often played a part in their lives. For example, one interviewee recalls her father often looking through a drawer filled with old photographs and some toys, but he never spoke about who the people were or who the toys had belonged to. Another recalls how she was taught by her parents to always have a pair of shoes by her bed, just in case there was a need to flee the home quickly (*Jerusalem Post* 2 July 2009).

As these children reached early adulthood in the 1970s, they began to collectively identify as survivors themselves. Fusing aspects of feminism, ethnic politics and humanistic psychology, these early pioneers 'urged their peers to break the silence about their familial legacy and make storytelling a vehicle for self-transformation, collective identification and social action (Stein 2009: 27). In this respect, it was the children of the camp survivors, not their parents, who were the main publicists of the Holocaust experience. The narration of their personal stories and the finding of shared experiences led to the adoption of the name 'second generation' and, in the process, personal experiences merged into collective identity.

According to Stein (2009), the movement's origins may have sprung from a conversation between five children of survivors (three women and two men) in 1975. They subsequently published the details of their conversation in a small readership Jewish magazine called *Response*, explaining that,

> Thirty years after World War II, the memory of the Holocaust lingers with us. For most survivors it has a daily effect. It also influences the thinking of the children of Holocaust survivors. Five of us, all in our twenties, got together in January 1975, to discuss this part of our heritage. We wanted to examine the extent to which our 'Weltanschauung' [worldview] is *determined* by the World War II experiences of our parents and families. Much of this is guesswork. We found that perspectives we thought were unique were in fact common to the whole group. More significantly, in our minds these perspectives were a result of the *direct* role the Holocaust played in our childhoods.
>
> (quoted in Stein 2009: 28, my emphasis)

For these offspring of camp survivors, the problem was that they 'were possessed by a history they had never lived' (Epstein 1988: 14). This attempt by the second generation to 'remember' events that they did not directly experience has been labelled 'post-memory', which is characterized as 'the experience of those who grow up dominated by narratives that preceded their birth' (Hirsch 1997: 22). The desire to 'know' a past that cannot be replicated, to re-member as a process not a recollection, has helped shape many children's Jewish identity around the shared trauma of the Holocaust. In a review of this genre, Eaglestone (2004: 81) notes how they 'articulate the complex intersection between identity, the past, memory, and culture and, centrally, they concern the process by which identification takes place and then is developed'.

Of course the Holocaust debate is multifaceted. Some point out that to portray all Jews as passive victims overlooks those who actively resisted Nazi persecution (Einwohner 2007). Others point out also that the binary of Jews as victims and Nazis as perpetrators overlooks those cases whereby survivors were badly exploited by fellow Jews in the years after the war (Wolf 2007). There are also those who are extremely critical of the way the experience of the war has become psychologized. For them, the aim was to publicize not psychologize the Holocaust, to emphasize social action rather than personal introspection. In this respect, there have been many positive developments in the way in which the children of Holocaust survivors articulated their experiences and shared them with others. Indeed, for some time after the end of the Second World War there was no collective experience known as the 'Holocaust'. Camp survivors' stories were, when discussed, more likely to be personal and familial in nature. Prior to the category of 'the Holocaust', most survivors referred to the events of 'the war' (Stein 2007). As Stein notes,

> Once coaxed by their children to speak, many survivors even-
> tually became more likely to share their experiences with others.
> By politicizing Holocaust victimhood, the second generation
> helped to bring the voices of survivors and their families into
> American public discourse.
>
> (Stein 2009: 48)

However, what is interesting is the way the Holocaust is felt to have been both a determining and direct factor in how the second generation viewed themselves and their experiences, as opposed to, say, having influenced them. Little recognition is given to how such present day subjectivity is shaped by a multitude of factors, not least, as we shall see in Chapter 5, by a cultural climate in which a therapeutic mode of understanding personal and social distress was coming to the fore. This is evidenced in the way an initial discussion among five people was a precursor to the 'second generation phenomenon' and the rise of what has been termed the 'Holocaust Industry' (Finkelstein 2000). The momentum with which a few people discussing their experiences can become a phenomenon, whereby the Holocaust has arguably become the symbolic marker of the twentieth century, indicates that it somehow tapped into the cultural zeitgeist. After all, how many other small groupings of people or social movements have sunk without a trace in the same period, no matter the legitimacy of what they were trying to achieve?

Such has been the plethora of books about the Holocaust that such writing can be described as being part of a narrative *genre* in its own right (Eaglestone 2004). Most such books are survivors' testimonies, others fictional accounts of the horrors of the period. Some books have even gone from the former to the latter, there being instances where the 'testimonial' is later found to be false, a work of fiction by the writer. One such account is that of Binjamin Wilkomirski (1996), whose book *Fragments* was initially well received and the author given elevated social status due to the 'horrors' he had 'experienced'. As Stefan Mächler notes,

> As a victim who could not have been more innocent and more ill-treated he was met with world-wide solidarity and boundless sympathy. As a person who never felt he belonged, he now found entry into a community of victims . . . The most important gain . . . was that he had found a meaningful story for an inexplicable and inaccessible past.
>
> (quoted in Eaglestone 2004: 125)

What is striking about the Wilkomirski affair is that most of those who have investigated it in depth are of the opinion that as a result of trauma and pain in his own life, Wilkomirski began to identify with the actual victims of the Holocaust. In a severe form of identification he took narcissistic possession of the Holocaust experience and also exploited the collective memory of it (Eaglestone 2004).

What such incidents show is the way in which the elevation of certain experiences within a given cultural moment can affect both past and present identification in the *process* of remembering. While such extreme accounts are rare, they do show the power of memory as a verb, as active rather than passive, and should alert us to the way less extreme forms of identification can occur within a cultural climate in which the sick role, victimhood and testimony-as-recognition have elevated status.

The expansion of trauma

The expansion of the concept of the 'survivor', while arguably most closely associated with the Holocaust, has less to do with the actual events of that period than with the way in which various social dynamics have seen the growth of the survivor identity as a social phenomenon from the 1970s onwards. One such dynamic was that of a process of psychologization and a therapeutically oriented form of feminism. The period following the Second World War saw the growth of a therapeutic society in both the USA and western Europe. Psychological theories moved from the clinic to the mainstream of society. The public expression of hitherto private secrets or hurt was increasingly held to be freeing and self-transforming. This discourse of psychological hurt and therapeutic remedy has become a powerful cultural paradigm within which people narrate their life histories and personal identity. Silence and reserve were transformed from being seen as reflective and stoical traits, to ones that indicated denial or repression. The recognition being sought is not primarily about according someone respect for their humanity, but of recognizing their past hurt, acknowledging the injuries inflicted on them by virtue of their individual or group difference, of 'feeling their pain'.

For feminists either suffering or working in the field of violence against women, the emerging focus on psychological harm caused by traumatic events proved extremely influential. Insights into the harmful effects of extreme situations such as war, torture, genocide and natural disasters (earthquakes, floods, famine, etc.) began to be applied to cases of interpersonal abuse. Such an approach was held to be progressive in that 'the trauma paradigm did not blame victims for their own victimization' which the previously dominant psychoanalytically informed explanations tended to do (Gilfus 1999: 1240). For Gilfus, there are several advantages to the application of trauma theory to the study of violence against women:

> First, it validates the psychological injury of acts such as adult sexual contact with children, or the psychological and physical abuse of an intimate partner, demonstrating that distress is often very severe and long lasting. Second, many of the forms of violence against women that are so painstakingly named and spoken out about can be incorporated within the trauma framework, helping us draw the parallels and connections between different types of violence. Women are often open to a trauma framework for understanding their pain and suffering and some of the more frightening after effects of victimization such as flashbacks and nightmares. It can be empowering to have a scientifically sound explanation that understands that one did not bring the violence upon oneself. Finally, trauma research has led to treatment interventions that offer relief from symptoms and are truly helpful to victims.
>
> (Gilfus 1999: 1241)

The 'everyday violence' suffered by women was equated with the trauma experienced by men in combat situations (Burstow 2003), and, as such, they are said to be suffering a form of post-traumatic stress disorder (PTSD). The expansion of the diagnostic category of PTSD is illustrative of the trend to medicalize human experience and normalize trauma. PTSD first appeared in the American Psychiatric Association's *Diagnostic and Statistical Manual of Mental Disorders* (DSM-III) in 1980, primarily concerned with the experiences of US soldiers on their return from the Vietnam War. Prior to this, DSM-II had subsumed the mental distress experienced during or after combat under standard psychiatric categories such as depression, psychosis or alcoholism (American Psychiatric Association (APA) 1968). It was not yet seen as a specific illness. However, as with much of psychiatry, the inclusion of PTSD as a mental disorder in DSM-III was more to do with politics than with advances in psychiatric epidemiology. It was influenced, to a not insubstantial degree, by the anti-war fervour within left-wing activism at the time, including anti-war psychiatrists and psychologists. As one sociologist put it:

> The struggle for *recognition* of PTSD by its champions was profoundly political, and displays the full range of negotiation, coalition formation, strategizing, solidarity affirmation, and struggle – both inside various professions and 'in the streets' – that define the term.
>
> (Scott 1990: 295, emphasis in original)

In other words, despite some strong objections from many within the psychiatric establishment to the inclusion of PTSD, the proponents were better organized, more politically motivated, active, and ultimately successful.

Here we see the influence of social movements and the politics of recognition discussed in earlier chapters. Those war veterans who advocated for the inclusion of PTSD in the DSM were seeking recognition for the psychological injury caused by the war. It would also indicate that in terms of the debate between Fraser and Honneth (2003), it is the latter's more psychologically orientated theoretical position that has most influenced the contemporary period. In addition, the recognition that is sought is not for past or present achievement, but for past or present victimization and the trauma that has resulted from it.

Of particular importance is the way in which the focus changed from the traumatized soldiers being seen as suffering an *abnormal*

reaction to their experiences to one where it is now considered normal
to experience such trauma. From this perspective, it is the failure to
recognize and treat the trauma that then results in PTSD. There is
little doubt that many individuals suffer extreme mental anguish as a
result of their wartime and indeed other experiences in their lives.
However, it is important to note that 'conceptions of our psychological states cannot be divorced from the social and political
processes' from which they arise and that 'what is at issue, in this case,
is the way normal and abnormal psychological adjustment has been
reconstructed around the "normality" of victimhood' (Lee 2001: 5).
This process can also be seen within international relations in the
changing way conflict situations are discussed and interventions
predicated. Whereas in previous times the focus of international
intervention in post-war situations was on material needs such as food
and shelter, more latterly it is a concern with the psychological state
of war-affected populations that is the focus of international policy.
In this respect trauma has replaced hunger in how the West portrays
the impact of wars and disasters in the South (Pupavac 2001). This
development can be seen closer to home in the way that the political
situation in Northern Ireland began to focus on reconciliation of past
hurt, the use of the language of empathy, and the tendency to view
politics as a form of therapeutic activity (Bean 2007).

Within both academia and professional practice the language of
trauma has been applied to describe the hurt experienced not only by
individuals but also by groups of people. African Americans, Jews,
Aborigines and many other native peoples see their collective histories
through the prism of trauma (e.g. Eyerman 2001). This second-hand
trauma, exemplified by the descendants of Holocaust survivors, is
now attributed to those affected as a result of the past trauma suffered
by increasing numbers of individuals and groups, and has been
termed 'transgenerational trauma' (Danieli 1998). A growing number
of mothers are said to suffer from 'birth trauma' due to the experience
of childbirth (*Guardian* 15 November 2010). Such groups and communities are now held to suffer from, or perhaps more accurately, be
bound together through a shared discourse of trauma.

Such developments tend to be viewed positively, with criticism
mainly directed at analyses where trauma theory often fails to fully
incorporate the political context within which the trauma takes place,
and for having a predominant medical orientation that individualizes a
socio-political problem. Analyses that focus on the psychological harm
suffered by the woman have also been criticized for reducing the
complexities of violence towards women to a form of psychopathology

(Gilfus 1999). Gilfus also notes how such a conflation can lead to a view that all forms of traumatic events cause psychological harm, something that risks reducing women to fragile victims adrift in a hostile world. However, it is worth pointing out that there is no consensus over the role of psychiatry in alleviating female trauma; while some view it as inherently problematic others largely accept a psychiatric paradigm albeit with some reservations (e.g. Herman 1992).

Many feminist theorists and activists, in their struggle against the pathologizing of trauma, sought, with some success, to reframe symptoms as coping skills (for example, in relation to self-harm), to accord significance to testimony, create more detailed and erudite critiques of mainstream psychiatry, and to normalize trauma over the 'normalcy' of safety (Burstow 2003). Indeed for Burstow and several other radicals, it is the very belief in and superior status accorded to 'normalcy' that is particularly problematic. From this perspective, the belief that the world is generally safe and benign and that therefore relations of trust should pertain is brought into question, as is the implication that the trauma survivor has a less realistic picture of the world than others. The rape survivor, for example, knows the world is a dangerous place, therefore they are said to have greater awareness than those who walk around with an aura of invincibility. Likewise, oppressed groups are only too aware that the world is not a safe environment (Burstow 2003). Indeed, from Glendenning's (1994) 'eco-feminist' perspective, the disjuncture between person and environment means that *everyone* associated with western civilization is traumatized, while Burstow (2003: 1308) sees the effects of oppression as extending even further to 'the earth itself'.

In order to arrive at such a conclusion, writers such as Burstow have to adopt a fundamentally anti-human outlook. Not only must all be cast as potential victims, but also, by extension, all interpersonal interactions need to be viewed through a prism of suspicion. Even her 'oppressed peoples' are disadvantaged by such a perspective. To fight for freedom from oppression requires collective solidarity, yet this is undermined by focusing on mistrust as the main paradigm through which to view societal and personal relations.

This tendency is unfortunate as, in many respects, there is much insight to be gained from the work of such theorists in terms of therapeutic understanding and practice issues for working with those people who have indeed been traumatized. However, by normalizing trauma they inadvertently undermine subjectivity and resilience among individuals and communities who become seen as requiring the expert intervention of the therapist to rehabilitate the community or group. The greatest irony is that despite the critiques of professional psychiatric power and ideology, the power of the psy-disciplines has, if anything, increased in recent years. And while writers such as Burstow are proud of the strand within feminism that has 'normalized trauma', such a process has influenced a climate where individual vulnerability rather than collective politics is emphasized.

From the Holocaust through feminism, deep ecology and its incorporation into wider discourse, the common framework is that of trauma. There is 'a sense that life is threatened by times of terror and helplessness in which conventional restraints, resources and forms of understanding are inadequate' (Gottlieb 1994).

Burstow argues that

> oppressed people are routinely worn down by the insidious trauma involved in living day after day in a sexist, racist, classist, homophobic, and ableist society: being ogled by men on the street, slaving long hours and for minimum wages in a fish processing plant, hearing racist innuendoes even from one's White allies.
>
> (Burstow 2003: 1296)

Burstow could be echoing the view of the UK government here. In recent years it has legislated to outlaw speech that others may find offensive, attempted to formalize interpersonal relationships via codes of conduct and harassment procedures, and instigated many therapeutic interventions to alleviate the psychological pain of the traumatized. 'Radical' proponents of the trauma paradigm fail to notice that their 'radical' view of people is shared by mainstream politicians.

For some (e.g. Herman 1992), psychological trauma is an affliction of the powerless individual although such individual vulnerability can have social roots, social disintegration being a factor in how individuals respond to traumatic events. As Summerfield (1996: 25) points out, 'psychological trauma is not like physical trauma: people do not passively register the impact of external forces (unlike, say, a leg hit by a bullet) but engage with them in an active and problem-solving way'. In this sense, the expansion of the concept of trauma is related to how we interpret our experiences and give meaning to our lives, and it would appear that the trauma framework has become increasingly influential, being no longer confined to the clinic it has now become embedded in popular culture. In 1994 there were fewer than 500 citations of the word 'trauma' in British newspapers; by the end of the decade the figure was over 5000 (cited in Furedi 2004).

The trauma paradigm's plasticity also means that it can be adopted by opposing camps. For example, in relation to abortion, many pro-choice activists argue that to give birth to an unwanted child, especially if the pregnancy was the result of rape, would be harmful to the woman's mental health. Similar arguments are also heard from pro-life activists who argue that future trauma awaits the woman who has an abortion, with some at the extreme end of the spectrum arguing that even in the case of abortion following incest or rape, 'abortion is equally destructive. Women report that they are suffering from the trauma of abortion long after the rape trauma has faded'. From this perspective the abortion is seen as 'the second rape' (Feminists for Life of America (FFL) 2008).

For many of these individuals and groups, the use of the specific term 'survivor' in relation to their trauma is an attempt to endow the individual or movement with moral authority, to allow their narrative to be accorded significance and their status enhanced. Indeed, while it may be an unwitting association by many, those groups claiming survivor status today seek their claims for legitimacy by an implicit elision between the horrors of the Holocaust and their own situation, no matter how mundane by comparison that may be.[2] Such 'historical analogies' are influenced by a therapeutic culture, or more precisely a therapeutically-informed feminism.

Breaking the silence: the battle for the past

Many survivor movements are engaged in what has been termed 'retrospective conflict'. They are contesting the dominant meaning attributed to past events with the aim of subverting dominant discourses and concomitant relations of power. In this sense, aspects of what has been termed a 'culture of survivorhood' can be utilized in order to affect not only a personal narrative but also socio-political change (DeGloma undated). For DeGloma,

> Survivor movements reframe past events, experiences, and social relationships in order to contest mainstream and entrenched perceptions of the past. By reframimg past events, they establish alternatives to the default meanings traditionally associated with them. The meaning attributed to the past then becomes the object of political struggle.
>
> (DeGloma undated: 5)

The survivor accounts of the past are themselves contested by what DeGloma calls *reactive conservative movements* that seek to preserve traditional images and views of the past. So, while a main focus of feminist critique was to highlight the often oppressive, violent and abusive nature of 'the family', for example by highlighting accounts of physical, sexual and psychological violence, the traditional conservative account would seek to preserve the view of it as the idyllic, harmonious realm of the happy heterosexual nuclear family, albeit one that is being undermined by modernity and decadent liberalism.

This polarization of a contested past is perhaps best crystallized in the 'recovered/false' memory debate in relation to childhood sexual abuse. Survivors attempt to show a continuation between the past and the present, where the individual's current mental distress is a result of the repression of said abuse, and where the memory of it has been recovered during therapy. In an insightful discussion of the false/recovered memory phenomenon, Burman (1996–97) links the debate to a generalized social anxiety in a fragmented postmodern world, where the very concepts of truth and certainty are thrown into question, and she notes how the discussion is framed in such a way that we are asked to choose between the polarities of either abused children or abusive therapists. In the process, complex social relations, anxieties over truth, history and futurity can be subsumed under the rubric 'abuse'.

In working with clients there are a range of theories which can be utilized, of which an interpersonal therapeutic relationship is important. In one-to-one relationships it is narrative accounts that are drawn on to explore the nature and meaning of clients' experiences. Consequently, the

> task is to open discursive spaces in which clients can develop their own interpretive story, that is, one that gives meaning to their experiences, and to understand how dominant discourses operate to suppress this story. In other words, it is about validating the client's entitlement to explain their lives in their own ways and in so doing assist their empowerment.
>
> (Dominelli 2002: 86)

This contrasts with some traditional therapeutic techniques where the aim is to 'reframe' the client's story in ways which attempt to assimilate it into the dominant discourses. Nevertheless, there is also a need to maintain a critical stance towards contemporary discursive representations of the self, in such a way as to allow the subject's position and contention to be challenged and probed rather than either summarily dismissed, as in traditional psychiatry, or uncritically accepted, as in much contemporary therapeutic work (Parker et al. 1995). Often, it is this complexity of memory, meaning and experience that gets lost when individual trauma, and recognition as dependent on it, becomes politicized.

For many childhood sexual abuse survivors, a key tactic has been to encourage other victims to disclose their ordeal also, to 'break the silence' surrounding a hitherto unacknowledged crime to achieve not only justice but also personal and societal change. For Alcoff and Gray (1993),

> Speaking out serves to educate the society at large about the dimensions of sexual violence and misogyny, to reposition the problem from the individual psyche to the social sphere where it rightfully belongs, and to empower victims to act constructively on our own behalf and thus make the transition from passive victim to active survivor.
>
> (Alcoff and Gray 1993: 261–262)

Similarly, a rape victim who went public about her experience states how she found her sanity when she found her voice (Ziegenmeyer 1992). This speaking out is seen as transgressive as it gives voice to those women and children who have been silenced by a dominant patriarchal society. Silencing tactics include charges of delusion, hysteria and madness as well as physical threats. Their opponents, often those accused of the abuse, seek to disconnect the present from the past by blaming the therapeutic process for implanting false memories. They reject any link between the past and present, a process described by Eviatar Zerubavel as 'mnemonic decapitations' (cited in DeGloma undated). As discussed above, Holocaust survivors were also encouraged, mainly by their children, to 'break the silence' about their ordeal, to speak out and in the process conserve the past and heal the present, as well as to counter the claims of Holocaust deniers. Likewise, psychiatric survivors are encouraged to 'come out' and identify as such in order to not only heal the individual but also to build the collective.

There are some reservations over the way in which such speaking out can be viewed as unproblematic. For example, Alcoff and Gray (1993) note five dangers of the confessional. First, it can reduce survivor speech to mere media commodity. Second, it can often focus attention on the victim and their state of mind rather than on the perpetrator. Third, for there to be a confessor there needs to be someone to confess to, yet this can render the speaker as subordinate to an expert who will interpret the precise accuracy and meaning of the confessor's words, thereby undermining the authority of the survivor. Fourth, it sets up binary structures, for example between experience and emotion which can be used against women by accusing them of being too sensitive and seeing abuse everywhere. Fifth, if speaking out is seen as a necessary tactic on the path to recovery, this can have a coercive, stigmatizing effect on those women, who, for whatever reason, choose to remain silent.

Nevertheless, 'Breaking the Silence' is seen as a prerequisite to recovery, speaking out the dominant motif within much social movement theory and individual self-conceptualization. According to Gilfus (1999), the survivor is seeking acknowledgement of their worth as a whole human being 'with a cultural and historical context, capable of expert knowledge, who is a subject in her or his own right, to be viewed through a lens of loving perception' (Gilfus 1999: 1253). To achieve this sense of worth, the post-silence utterance in and of itself is not enough. It must be accorded positive affirmation. The verbalization of past trauma and identification as a 'survivor' represents a demand for recognition; the past abuse is seen as more hurtful because society fails to acknowledge that it has taken place.

The issue of public recognition for past trauma surfaced in relation to the debate over the issue of satanic ritual abuse (SRA) and survivor's testimonies. This topic came to public attention during the 1980s and 1990s. For some supporters of the reality of the victims' testimonies, the absence of evidence, or indeed the incredulity of the testimonial, is not a reason for disbelief. On the contrary the more unbelievable the survivors' story, the more reason to suspect it as having some firm basis in truth. From this perspective, the more unbelievable the account is, the more we should believe it. The more an identity is dissociative, the more we should believe that the uttered experiences of abuse are true (Cook and Kelly 1997).

Following this argument, Cook and Kelly (!997) draw similarities with the Nazi Holocaust, where there was a belief that the sheer scale of the atrocities would mean that the world would not believe them, and also that it was the testimonies of camp survivors that exposed the horrors endured within them. Such an argument is flawed in two ways. First, there were also eye-witness accounts of the camps from liberators and documentary footage of the malnourishment of the survivors. Second, it is not reasonable to compare the systematic slaughter, based on ideologies of racial superiority and eugenics, of over six million Jews, to the isolated and geographically distant cases cited in SRA testimonies.

The self as reference point

Such is the sensitivity to criticism of writers such as Cook and Kelly (1997) that those who question the extent of ritualized abuse are accused of undermining the experiences of all women and children who have experienced sexual abuse. However, of particular interest is that their most pressing concern is that to question accounts of such abuse fails to accord the women due recognition. To question their subjective experience is to withhold respect. This highlights one of the dangers inherent in the prevalence of contemporary therapeutic discourse, whereby the self becomes the only reference point, with the social dimension correspondingly downgraded.

The impact of therapeutic sensibilities on feminism was profound as many in the movement turned inward towards the self in the pursuit of a revolution from within. Illouz (2008) argues that it was a discursive alliance between feminism and a therapeutic culture that helped pave the way for such things as the confessional talk show, the growth of the recovery movement and the expansion of psychiatric diagnostic categories. As Stein (2009) notes:

> Across the nation, communities of alcoholics, teenage children of alcoholics, women who 'love too much', and victims of sexual abuse formed collective identities based on common suffering, encouraging their participants to publicly acknowledge their injuries. These therapeutic social movements, operating on the border between the personal and the public spheres, made selfhood a narrative to be shared publicly.
>
> (Stein 2009: 30)

This focus on the self and its needs is a common theme throughout the wider survivor phenomenon. In this respect, the self becomes the key, if not the only reference point. Subjective experience overrides objective analysis. In a sense historians have become marginalized in relation to the investigation of the past, the interrogation and reflection on the past being ceded to the various 'psy-professionals' – psychiatrists, psychologists, psychoanalysts – and also to individual recollection. For example, Stein (2009: 46) notes that 'the authority of professional historians was being challenged by the growing influence of non-professional witnesses – namely, Holocaust survivors and their descendants'. A similar concern is expressed by Cesarani (2001) in his belief that we live in an 'epoch preoccupied by memory and memorialization', a 'confessional culture' in which individual historical narratives are accorded the highest priority (Cesarani 2001: 7). This is problematic because memories or personal narratives are not only individual but collective in nature. Memory is not recalled in the same way as the replaying of a videoed event. Its interpretation, and the significance attached to the interpretation are socially, culturally and politically embedded.

Although many view identification as a survivor as a positive move, an agentic action as opposed to that of passive victim, there have been many critics who argue that the survivor phenomenon represents a cult of victimhood. In relation to Holocaust survivors, Novick (1999) noted how,

> The cultural icon of the strong, silent hero is replaced by the vulnerable and verbose antihero. Stoicism is replaced as a prime value by sensitivity. Instead of enduring in silence, one lets it all hang out. The voicing of pain and outrage is alleged to be 'empowering' as well as therapeutic.
>
> (Novick 1999: 9)

In addition, actual survivors can be criticized for refusing to speak out about their experiences. Instead of such silence and reserve being seen as an act of strength, a display of fortitude, it is likely to be viewed as a form of repression or denial. In such a process the very refusal to embrace the victim identity is both stigmatized and pathologized.

Although Alcoff and Gray (1993: 269) inform us that 'the point of contention between dominant and survivor discourses is not over the determination of truth but over the determination of the statable', their discussion leaves little doubt that to dispute 'survivor' speech is to do a grave injustice not only to that individual, but also to all survivors. They detail 'the method of anonymous accusation' employed by female students at Brown University in the USA in 1990, where the women began writing the names of rapists on the bathroom walls, which caused 'great consternation for the named perpetrators'. Favouring such strategies may 'minimize the dangers of speaking out for survivors yet maximize the disruptive potential of survivor outrage' (Alcoff and Gray 1993: 286), but it also risks vigilante justice and false accusations. In effect, the refusal to believe is stigmatized, meaning that 'the accuser is accorded monopoly over some transcendental truth' (Furedi 1997: 79). The usefulness of such a strategy in terms of individual therapeutic catharsis is questionable. As a political measure it is deeply problematic, as are the implications for the judicial process of anonymous accusations.

This privileging of victim testimony is also apparent within social policy in the UK. For example, in relation to race, the Macpherson Report into the killing of Stephen Lawrence (Macpherson 1999) recommended that a racist incident be defined as such if that is how it was perceived by the victim. Guidance to all staff working within the National Health Service makes it clear that it is for the 'victim' to determine whether they have been harassed, abused or bullied (General Whitley Council (GWC) 2000).

Power and the confessional

Following the death of her husband Jonathan, killed by a psychiatric patient inside a London tube station in December 1992, Jayne Zito set up the Zito Trust, an organization which had the aim of high-lighting the failings of community care and calling for more restrictions to be placed on former patients.[3] For Jayne, the campaign also had a more personal therapeutic aspect in allowing her a space to talk about her experience and feelings. By campaigning she felt she could talk about how she felt and work through her feelings as she did so.

Others similarly use media coverage as a therapeutic outlet for their grief. Bookshops are filled with 'misery memoirs' that detail the author's past abuse, while television talk shows such as those hosted by Oprah Winfrey, Trisha Goddard and Jeremy Kyle encourage their guests to disclose their most personal and traumatic experiences for public consumption. While these shows tend to be aimed at a lower working class demographic, more middle class radio listeners are provided with a not dissimilar service by way of such programmes as Radio 4's *In the Psychiatrist's Chair*. Posters advertising the services of helplines and services proliferate. Far from being viewed as episodes in life to be ashamed of, or at the very least to keep quiet about, today 'the ability to survive potentially destructive experiences like drug abuse or a psychological syndrome has been reinterpreted as an act of bravery worthy of our applause' (Furedi 2004: 43). To 'survive' is now held to be a source of pride, a triumph in and of itself.

In contemporary society, the confessional is no longer confined within the church or the analyst's consulting room. It has gone public. Private pain increasingly requires a public forum for its expression, acknowledgement and therapeutic soothing of the psyche. More and more people pursue personal healing via public exposure. In this respect the survivor phenomenon is part of, and has become institutionalized and politicized in, a climate in which a therapeutic mode of personal understanding, of psychological vulnerability, dominates the political and public sphere to such an extent that to resist it is itself seen as a marker of a flawed psychology. In contemporary western culture, a victim identity accords the individual a degree of moral authority.

Without doubting the barriers that people experiencing past or current abuse can still confront, contemporary culture is far more amenable to disclosures of abuse than in the past. However, this is not wholly progressive. The art of confession takes place within certain parameters which can replicate power differentials in the very process of ostensibly undermining them.

If the ability to speak out is empowering for the individual concerned and also for social justice, the wider survivor narrative can be co-opted within a framework that can be just as disempowering for the individuals concerned. As Foucault (1972) noted, the ability to formulate speech and to have it listened to, is an important site of conflict permeated by a power/knowledge nexus. In contrast to the days in which abuse victims were effectively silenced in society, contemporary culture is far more receptive to stories of trauma. So, while the act of speaking out changes power dynamics this is not always to the benefit of the speaker. In the modern equivalent of the confessional, namely the therapeutic encounter, the confessor will tell his or her story to the interviewer and the audience, and often there will be a psychiatrist or psychologist present whose role is to interpret what the speaker has said and tell us its 'true meaning'. In this process, far from being the active subject, the speaker is reduced to an object of expert analysis. The media can also focus on the sensationalist aspects of stories, offering up survivors' accounts more for audience titillation than serious discussion. In order to be believed, the role of victim must be played, for example crying for the television or newspaper camera. The identity offered up for public consumption is one of suffered trauma; it is a therapeutic identity that is required for the achievement of public recognition today.

Conclusion

The move from the old to the new social movements entailed the adoption of a politics of recognition, where there was an emphasis on the hurt caused to the integrity of the self by the withholding of recognition. Increasingly, the form of recognition that was demanded was recognition of survival of past trauma, affirmation of a psyche further damaged by the hitherto failure of society to recognize individual or group suffering. These developments were influential in the rise of the 'survivor' phenomenon. From an initial concern with extreme experiences such as the Nazi Holocaust, the number of experiences that could be 'survived' has proliferated, with many more groups and individuals emphasizing their identity and status by use of the survivor suffix, whether victim of an extreme experience or less severe form of distress.

This expansion of the concept of trauma survivor has taken place in a cultural climate that is increasingly amenable to psychological explanations for individual and social problems, and also where conceptual boundaries are blurred to the extent that to speak of *the* (Nazi) Holocaust (with a capital H) can be seen as failure to recognize many other holocausts.

It is important to recognize the way in which the trauma victim discourse confuses the reality of the Holocaust with subjective responses to it. This discourse then uses the subjective response as a way to understand the real event, which risks depoliticizing the Holocaust by reducing it to a traumatic, subjective, self-referential discourse. The discursive process itself then plays a part in the creation of the subjective experience as a new kind of reality for those involved; the individual is 'traumatized' and they do feel vulnerable.

The demand for recognition increasingly necessitated recognition not for what the individual or group had done, but rather, on what had been done to her/them. Influenced by a form of therapeutic feminism, campaigners were concerned to give the traumatized 'a voice'. Consequently, more and more people were encouraged to 'speak out' and 'break the silence' around abusive relationships whether of a personal or wider societal nature.

It is perhaps no surprise that in a political climate where the old ways of articulating and expressing alienation and dissent no longer have much societal resonance, people look to other ways to give meaning to their experiences. In this respect, the normalization of trauma and the promotion of the fragile self are best analysed not as a psychological issue but as a historical and political one.

To further develop this line of argument the next chapter takes a look at one specific survivor identity, that of the 'psychiatric survivor', in order to illustrate the historical specificity of both the identity and such a way of viewing the world and one's place within it.

Notes

1 Exodus International's website is http://exodusinternational.org
2 Betty Friedan uses such a rhetorical elision in her 1963 book *The Feminine Mystique* (Friedan 1986) when she refers to the domestic household as a 'comfortable concentration camp' for women. She later regretted the use of such an analogy. In an interesting article on Holocaust consciousness, Fermaglich (2003) argues that while an exaggerated and flawed analogy, Friedan's use of it demonstrates that American Jewish intellectuals were aware of the horrors of the Holocaust earlier than many historians have recognized.
3 The Zito Trust was influential in the campaign to introduce community treatment orders for psychiatric patients, and which were indeed included in the Mental Health Act 2007. Having achieved its aims, it has now disbanded.

4　Surviving psychiatry

One of the most recent 'new social movements' has been that of the mental health user/survivor groupings. These range from those who are happy to accept having their opinion taken seriously by the psychiatric and related professionals but who otherwise accede to their authority, to those who want more of a partnership, and yet others who reject the very existence of mental illness and therefore do not accept psychiatry as having any form of expertise in understanding or alleviating mental distress.

As we shall see, opposition to psychiatric theory and practice has as long a history as psychiatry itself. However, in relation to contemporary user-led groups, the closure of the asylum system and the concomitant move to care in the community has been the major structural and policy factor that has influenced the formation of mental health patients as a *social* movement. If you are confined in an institution, your ability to interact with wider society is somewhat constrained.

It is difficult to say with precision what was the main driver behind the closure of the large scale psychiatric institutions and move to community care. A variety of factors have been cited by some and criticized by others, such as the discovery of anti-psychotic medication that appeared to alleviate many patients' symptoms, the fiscal crisis of the 1970s, the critiques of the 'anti-psychiatry' movement, and the publication of reports documenting the mistreatment of patients within the closed walls of the total institutions. It was most likely a combination of all of these and other complex dynamics that resulted in the change of policy towards the inmates of the old asylums.

Whatever the reason, the move to community care is obviously of great importance as a catalyst for the contemporary visibility and voice of the mental health user movement. In this chapter I look at some of the intellectual critiques of psychiatry that have influenced the current situation, in particular the contribution of those subject to psychiatric authority; the patients, consumers and survivors of mental health services themselves. As well as drawing on such 'voices', the wider discourse in which they are articulated, expressed and interpreted is linked to ideological, social and political change. Insights from the preceding chapters also serve as a prism through which to locate contemporary developments and views of the psychiatric subject, whether that is as a patient, consumer or survivor. Finally, I discuss some implications of the adoption of a survivor identity.

Anti-psychiatry

The power of psychiatry should not be underestimated. It is able to categorize, diagnose and treat those deemed mad, a power achieved not only through its medical position as arbiter between normal and abnormal behaviour, but also by a legal system that gives certain psy-professionals the power to detain and medicate certain people against their will. Despite, or indeed because of such power, it has faced much criticism; from its inception through to the present day, its theories, practices and societal role have been subject to much critique. For example, by viewing insanity as a disease and not as punishment from God for sin or immoral ways, the new found discipline found itself in conflict with the Church. It also posed a threat to the very fabric of Christian thought because,

> In traditional Christian thought the mind was closely associated with the soul and assumed to be, like the soul, immortal and impervious to disease. If, on the other hand, insanity was a physical disorder of the brain, as eighteenth-century physicians usually insisted, and the mind simply the brain functioning, as some materialists maintained . . . then the brain, mind, and the soul as well were subject to disease and death; therefore the Christian concept of the immortal soul was invalid.
>
> (Dain 1994: 416)

The role of psychiatry in legitimizing oppressive social relations has also been extensively documented. Drapetomania was a nineteenth century 'mental disorder' said to afflict black slaves who fled captivity. With slavery justified on the basis that it was part of the natural order, then those slaves not content with their 'natural' position were deemed to be disordered. In the former Soviet Union, it was not uncommon for dissidents to be labelled mentally ill and detained in institutions. It was not until 1974 that the American Psychiatric Association declassified homosexuality as a mental disorder. In addition, numerous psychological, psychoanalytical, sociological and philosophical perspectives have criticized much psychiatric theory and practice. Further examples of both explicit and implicit racist assumptions have also been highlighted (e.g. Browne 1990; Fernando 2010), as has the role of psychiatry in upholding problematic gender roles and the construction of madness as a female malady (e.g. Chesler 1972; Showalter 1987).

The early twentieth century also saw challenges to mainstream psychiatry from the philanthropic reform movements such as the Central Association for Mental Welfare (founded in 1913), the National Council for Mental Hygiene (founded in 1922) and the Child Guidance Council (founded in 1927). Other professionals such as psychologists and social workers, often influenced by Freudian theory, also attempted to stake their claim to be best positioned to alleviate mental distress. However, the period following the Second World War saw the beginning of a more sustained attack on the tenets of psychiatry from a group of writers frequently seen as being at the forefront of what was termed the 'anti-psychiatry' movement. These writers, many of whom worked within the system, were a major source of intellectual and therapeutic inspiration for the contemporary mental health user/survivor movement. They not only challenged the medical and ethical claims of psychiatry but also implemented new and radical ways of working with the mentally distressed.

Discussion of the 'anti-psychiatry' movement usually refers to the work of such writers as R.D. Laing, David Cooper and Thomas Szasz, all of whom were practising psychiatrists or psychoanalysts and who challenged the very basis of mainstream psychiatric theory and practice. For Szasz (1961), what are termed mental illnesses or diseases are not due to faulty physicochemical processes but are, in reality, problems in living. The mind, like the economy, can be sick only in a metaphorical not literal sense. Mental illness as akin to a medical illness is therefore a myth. Szasz (1961) should not be misread as suggesting that personal troubles and distress do not exist, but, instead, that what we term mental health and mental illness are but new words for describing moral values and judgements, a form of secular ethics.[1] Viewing them through a medical framework is therefore to deny the ethical, personal and social conflicts from which they arise. Szasz's libertarianism and objection to the oppression of institutional psychiatry sits well with contemporary campaigns such as those against electro-convulsive therapy and community treatment orders. He is still active today, his protests against psychiatric coercion still appearing in 'anti-psychiatry' publications (e.g. Szasz 2010).

Laing was influenced by the existentialism of Jean-Paul Sartre. He rejected psychiatric classifications, refusing to use medical categories with his patients. Laing believed that it was necessary to try to understand the patient's reality, using existential phenomenology in order 'to articulate what the other's "world" is and ways of being in it' (Laing 1965: 25). He also believed that the psychotic condition may have some positive elements in that the 'schizophrenic' may have insight into the human condition not available to the sane, as 'the cracked mind of the schizophrenic may *let in* light that does not enter the intact minds of the many sane people whose minds are closed' (Laing 1965: 27, emphasis in original). From this perspective, society was seen as irrational, madness as a rational response to an insane society. Another influential writer was Marius Romme, a Dutch psychiatrist whose work has inspired several contemporary user/survivor groups, for example the Hearing Voices Network, Asylum Associates and Psychology Politics Resistance, and who can often be found contributing to radical publications and conferences.

In addition, Goffman's (1961) work on asylums exposed the dehumanizing effects of incarceration and the way in which the person became 'the patient', a process that led to the degradation of the self. Goffman (1961) detailed how on entering the institution the person went through a 'degradation ceremony'; being stripped of their own clothes and given uniform hospital clothing, and encouraged by staff to disown their previous life and adapt to the new environment. In short, they were stripped of their previous identity and became 'the patient'. A more historical account is given by Foucault (1967), whose *Madness and Civilisation* details the way medicine and psychiatry achieved its dominant position as the 'expert' voice in the categorization and treatment of those deemed 'mad'. This objectification of personhood is a frequent focus of complaint by those with a psychiatric diagnosis as they find that many professionals and the general public view them through the prism of the diagnosis. 'Once a schizophrenic, always a schizophrenic' is the perception (Barham and Hayward 1995), and many rightly object to this deterministic viewpoint with its lack of belief in people's capacity to change and transcend their problems.

Although all these influential writers have the same object of critique, it would be a mistake to view them as representing one body of thought or political opinion. Laing and Cooper, for example, were influenced by Marxist dialectics and revolutionary politics. Szasz was a libertarian supporter of free market capitalism who viewed Laing in particular as being 'a preacher of and for the "soft" underbelly of the New Left' (Szasz 1976: 5). They rarely collaborated. Laing claims to have met Szasz on only three occasions, and while Laing and Cooper are frequently spoken about in the same breath, to the extent that at times the work of one can be misattributed to the other and vice versa, they collaborated only occasionally. Laing claims that they had 'friendly respect for each other' but that the type of therapeutic work they were doing within their respective therapeutic communities, Kingsley Hall for Laing, Villa 21 for Cooper, were incompatible (Mullan 1995: 195).

Given the disagreements within the theories and practices of those antagonistic towards psychiatry, from various sources at various points in history, it should be clear that the term 'anti-psychiatry' should not be read as implying a homogenous grouping of either people or ideology. On the contrary, it

> is an amorphous concept that has never had any fixed meaning. It has changed over time and in connection with religious, legal, political, and social concerns as well as changes in psychiatry and the mental hospital . . . Anti-psychiatry can therefore be defined only as sets of attitudes, opinions, and activities antagonistic to psychiatry.
>
> (Dain 1994: 425)

Nevertheless, the combined work of these writers although largely ignored within the psychiatric profession at the time, was extremely influential within the broader cultural climate and, as we discuss below, continues to resonate among psychiatry's latter day opponents. The wider cultural resonance of the anti-psychiatry critique can be seen in the 1975 film *One Flew Over the Cuckoo's Nest*, in which the psychiatric institution and professionals are viewed as oppressive and damaging to the well-being of the inmates, with the feigned madness of the film's main character McMurphy, played by Jack Nicholson, seen as liberating and enlightening, a free spirit confined and gradually destroyed by a brutal regime. The pop star David Bowie's album *Aladdin Sane* (A lad insane) was also influenced by the cultural critique and silencing of mental distress, and also by family experience.[2]

If the ideas of the anti-psychiatry 'movement' resonated with a wider culture increasingly challenging the status quo and relations of power, within traditional psychiatry such views were more readily treated with disdain. Indeed, the term 'anti-psychiatry' can actually be used against user/survivors as professionals attempt to reclaim psychiatric hegemony. As Campbell has noted, anti-psychiatry 'has become a slogan that is routinely used by traditional mental health workers to denigrate and dismiss ideas that threaten their expert world-view and status' (Campbell 1996: 221).

In addition, the anti-psychiatry movement was not a user movement; it was dominated by professionals, many of whom were themselves psychiatrists. As Barnes and Bowl (2001: 32) pointed out, 'the voices claiming the right to re-define the nature of the experience of schizophrenia were not those who had been assigned the diagnosis, but academics and practitioners'. In this respect, the mental health *user* movement is a relatively recent phenomenon originating in both the UK and USA in the early 1970s. With the increased focus on civil rights from the 1950s onwards and the challenge to the withholding of them to certain groups, for example black people, women, gays and lesbians, and more recently people with disabilities, it may be the case that such concerns and self-mobilizations would eventually reach psychiatric patients themselves, for, as Campbell (1996: 219) notes, 'Madpersons may be mad, but they are not stupid. Inevitably, we would recognize and act upon the discrepancy between being promised that we were the same as everyone else and being treated as burdensome, dangerous, inferior aliens'.

The rise of the user/survivor movement

The late 1950s and 1960s saw 'some early indications of an emerging user voice' in the UK, albeit of a marginal nature (Crossley 1998: 482). In the USA, Chamberlin (1990) cites the first sustainable movement being the Insane Liberation Front, formed in 1970 in Portland, Oregon. In the UK, the same period saw the formation of the Scottish Union of Mental Patients, a 27-strong organization, and which developed more comprehensively with the formation of the Mental Patients Union (MPU) in 1973. The impetus for the formation of the MPU was the proposed closure of Paddington Day Hospital, a therapeutic community in London, a move opposed by the MPU.

Of course, individual and groups of patients opposed to the way psychiatry treated them go back much further than the 1970s. Coleman (1996) identifies the 1600s when the patients of Bethlem wrote a petition to the House of Lords complaining about their treatment and living conditions. Accounts by individuals critical of their treatment by psychiatry have also been traced back to this period. However, while it is obvious that individual protest does not constitute a social movement, neither does a one-off collective protest. The Bethlem petition may have been patient (user) led but this does not constitute a social movement. It may have had the potential to become a movement, but as Crossley (1999) points out, such instances are better described as constituting 'sporadic resistance'. In contrast, a social movement requires 'a degree of spatial-temporal extension and continuity' that was not evident in earlier protests. To constitute a social movement, a collective or activity must have 'a durable and dispersed culture of resistance and the mechanisms of reproduction which perpetuate and transmit it' (Crossley 1999: 652).

Today, there is most certainly such a durable and dispersed culture, albeit one that is also fluid and malleable. MINDLINK, a space for user-led activity within the mental health charity MIND, established in 1988, had a membership of over 700 within four years (Barnes and Bowl 2001). Fewer than 12 'psychiatric survivors' organizations existed in the UK in 1985, yet ten years later there were about 350 or more such groups at a local, regional and national level (Campbell 1996). In 2001, over 200 psychiatric 'survivor workers' attended the First National Conference of Survivor Workers UK in Manchester, and it was reported that a similar number had to be turned away due to the hall not being big enough to accommodate them. Those in and outside the conference were people who had current or past mental health problems and who now worked in a variety of organizations including within the mental health profession. The UK Advocacy Network (UKAN), formed in 1991with the main aim of providing training and support to local advocacy groups had, by 1998, over 220 groups affiliated to the network (Barnes and Bowl 2001). In the USA it has been estimated that there are approximately 7467 mental health mutual support groups, self-help organizations and consumer-operated services (Goldstrom et al. 2006), and that 60 per cent of ex-patient groups considered themselves to be psychiatric survivors (Everett 1994).

There is also a European Network of former Users and Survivors of Psychiatry, a World Network of former Users and Survivors of Psychiatry (Snow 2002) and a Recovery Movement, which similarly developed out of the civil rights movements of the 1960s and 1970s. The Recovery Movement was, and indeed still is, concerned with challenging the notion that people with psychiatric diagnoses are unable to recover from their difficulties, believing that such negative beliefs lead to little work being done on people's ability to improve their condition and which therefore contribute to a form of 'learned helplessness' (Allott 2000; see also Deegan 1992).

Testimonies, both written and oral, from people who have experienced and/or recovered from mental distress have helped to publicize the personal meanings behind diagnostic labels, as well as allowing the passing on of successful coping strategies for managing the crisis, and highlighting some abuses suffered by people while within the psychiatric system (e.g. Chamberlin 1978; Deegan 1992).

International coalitions of similar groups often share common goals against what they describe as human rights violations in the psychiatric system such as electroconvulsive therapy, forced medication/drugging, confinement without trial and the influence of the pharmaceutical industry on psychiatry (Chamberlin 1990). Breggin (1991) estimated that the pharmaceutical industry provided between 15 and 20 per cent of the American Psychiatric Association's total yearly budget. More recently in the USA, a study found that the drug companies had funded a programme that was campaigning for assertive community treatment – for treatment read medication (cited in Capstone Report 2001).

Snow (2002) argues that the UK Conference of Survivor Workers held in 2001 would have been unlikely to have been convened a decade earlier and would have been inconceivable in the early 1980s. Such a development indicates a growth in the confidence of many who suffer or have suffered mental distress to go public with their experiences. For some attendees, survivor workers can be revolutionary agents of change. Such a view may be misplaced optimism or general hyperbole, but the fact that the conference was sponsored by both the Manchester Health Authority and the Northwest NHS Regional Office is also testament to the growing influence of user/survivor groups within mainstream mental health provision. I use the word *influence* because, as one contributor to the conference points out, influence is not the same as power (Snow 2002). It may also be the case that the government, policymakers, health and related professions lack confidence regarding the legitimacy and/or efficacy of their role, and therefore seek to achieve some form of flattery and authority by such user associations.

Some specific groups emerge and dissolve over the years but the movement itself continues. For example, Survivors Speak Out formed in 1986, and, the following year, produced a 'Charter of Needs and Demands' which summarised its position as shown in the box:

Survivors speak out conference 1987 charter of needs and demands
The national conference of psychiatric system survivors held on September 18–20 1987 unanimously agreed the following list of needs and demands:

1. That mental health service providers recognize and use people's first hand experience of emotional distress for the good of others.
2. Provision of refuge, planned and under the control of survivors of psychiatry.
3. Provision of free counselling for all.
4. Choice of services including self-help alternatives.
5. A Government review of services, with recipients sharing their views.
6. Provision of resources to implement self-advocacy for all users.
7. Adequate funding for non-medical community services, especially crisis intervention.
8. Facility for representation of users and ex-users of services on statutory bodies. Including Community Health Councils, Mental Health Tribunals and the Mental Health Act Commission.
9. Full and free access to all personal medical records.
10. Legal protection and means of redress for all psychiatric patients.
11. Establishment of the democratic right of staff to refuse to administer any treatment without risk of sanction or prejudice.
12. The phasing out of electro-convulsive therapy and psychosurgery.
13. Independent monitoring of drug use and its consequences.
14. Provision for all patients of full written and verbal information on treatments, including adverse research findings.
15. An end to discrimination against people who receive, or have received, psychiatric services: with particular regard to housing, employment, insurance etc.

(http://studymore.org.uk/mpu.htm#EdaleCharter)

Survivors Speak Out (SSO) had some success in facilitating the growing survivor movement, holding conferences, spreading the word regarding self-advocacy and producing publications on self-harm, eating disorders and a comparison between user/survivor activism in the USA, UK and Europe. It did not, however, have agreed policies that it actively campaigned around, with the exception of the ultimately unsuccessful attempt to derail the proposals to extend compulsory powers under the Mental Health Act. Its influence waned towards the end of the 1990s and, while not formally wound up, SSO no longer plays an active part in the survivor movement (Campbell 2010). However, the demise of a particular organisation does not mean the end of the movement as a whole; self help groups have grown in the intervening period since SSO's heyday, most notably the Hearing Voices Network which organized the Second World Hearing Voices Congress on 2–4 November 2010. And all of SSO's charter demands are still advocated by various individuals or groups within the mental health field, partly, but not solely due to many members of SSO now belonging to other campaign groups. Indeed,

> in terms of membership, it is possible to draw a direct lineage from the MPU through to PROMPT (Protection of the Rights of Mental Patients in Treatment/Therapy) to CAPO (Campaign against Psychiatric Oppression) to current groups like Survivors Speak Out, the Self Harm Network and the Hearing Voices Network.
>
> (Spandler 2006: 65–66)

These groups are more interested in the content and meaning of the voices heard rather than seeing them as auditory hallucinations symptomatic of 'schizophrenia'. Other services are available from such organizations such as advocacy, drop-in facilities and social activities. They have established useful and practical protocols to improve the treatment of those who need psychiatric services, for example the introduction of 'crisis cards', which can be carried by people who may be susceptible to a mental health crisis but who are unable to articulate their problem and needs at such times. The card could carry details of medication prescribed (or wanted), allergies, as well as contact details for friends, family or professionals in case of emergency.

Other organizations, whose members may belong to several simultaneously and who also work with like-minded professionals, include Asylum Associates and Psychology Politics Resistance (PPR). These groups are linked by the quarterly magazine *Asylum: The Magazine for Democratic Psychiatry*. The magazine incorporates the newsletter of PPR, an organization founded in 1994 as 'a network of people – both psychologists and non-psychologists – who are prepared to oppose the abusive uses of psychology' (Parker et al. 1995: 143), and who had by 2001 effectively taken control of *Asylum* magazine (Parker 2001).

The above presents a mere snapshot of some of the user/survivor groupings, networks, affiliations and campaigns. My intention is not to provide an ethnographic account of user/survivor groups; for those wanting more detail, the work of writers such as Campbell (1996), Crossley (2006) and Spandler (2006) will prove useful. My main intention is to view the growth of such movements within the wider cultural and intellectual environment from which they emerged. It is to these influences and their implications that we now turn.

Patient, consumer, user or survivor: what's in a name?

The turn to discourse in contemporary social theory is a significant development within the field of mental health where terminology is extremely important, since the battle over signification has consequences for those signified. When a psychiatrist gives someone a diagnosis such as 'schizophrenia', that individual's social and legal status changes: the very process of iteration creates that which it names. This can lead to positive outcomes, such as enabling access to much needed health or social services. It can give a name and meaning to experiences, allowing the individual, their family, friends and carers to locate their difficulties within a framework that offers both diagnosis and prognosis. However, this comes at a price. The attribution of a psychiatric framework to personal and social difficulties can individualize and medicalize social problems, and can lead to the objectification of the subject who gets lost behind the diagnosis. The recipient of the diagnosis also finds that their status in society changes. Now categorized as mentally ill, the now patient loses many of the rights of citizenship that most of us take for granted.

In this respect, Beresford et al. (2000) are wrong to argue that 'there is little difference between having a physical impairment and being a survivor of the psychiatric system' due to both having few rights effectively enshrined in law and both being 'stereotyped as defective, dependent, tragic and threatening' (Beresford et al. 2000: 210). This may be true to an extent but there is one important difference that affects the mental patient and not those who are solely physically impaired. The former can, subject to certain conditions being met, be detained under the Mental Health Act against their will. This loss of liberty is not necessarily on the grounds of what the individual has done; it can be justified on the basis of what the psychiatrist and related professionals think they might do in the future, or solely because it is felt that it will be beneficial to their health. The right to refuse medical treatment can also be lost, and with the introduction of community treatment orders (CTOs) in the Mental Health Act 2007, such enforced treatment now extends beyond the walls of the hospital and into the patient's lifeworld post discharge. Whether done with the best of intentions or not, such measures inevitably reduce the subject's status, rendering him or her as under increased professional power and control. Indeed, ten times as many CTOs were issued in the first year they were available as an option for professionals than had been forecast, an indication that they are being used more for the benefit of risk averse professionals, who fear something going wrong (for example a serious incident involving a patient who had stopped taking their prescribed medication), rather than for the therapeutic benefit of their patients (Mental Health Foundation (MHF) 2010).

In attempting to redress this power imbalance one significant area of struggle has been over terminology. Much discussion has taken place as to whether those who use or are subject to mental health services are patients, consumers or survivors. The choice reflects the individual's attitude to, and relation with, mainstream psychiatry. In general, the 'patient' is seen as a passive recipient of psychiatry, someone who accepts that they are ill and submits, to a greater or lesser degree, to the authority of the psychiatrist (Barnes and Shardlow 1997). The 'consumer' (a term more popular in the USA but which is becoming more common in the UK) is held to be one who chooses their care from a range of options, someone who will actively negotiate with mental health services as to which is the most suitable package of care to meet their needs. The consumer may challenge psychiatric knowledge but they ultimately accept and accede to it (Speed 2006). The term 'survivor' in relation to mental health can have different meanings. It can be

> intended as a more broad term to include people who have experienced mental or emotional distress, whether or not they have used mental health services. However, 'survivor' may also be used politically to refer to people who have survived mental health services and/or treatments; in this sense it is shorthand for psychiatric system survivor.
>
> (Faulkner 2004: 2)

For survivors, it is not only their mental distress that they claim to have survived but also the psychiatric system itself. In this sense, they see psychiatry as contributing to, rather than alleviating their problems. They also reject the medical model and psychiatric authority, believing that they have overcome psychiatric oppression and therefore wish to maintain a distance between themselves and the dominant psychiatric framework (Chamberlin 1990).

The rejection of the medical paradigm is endorsed by many survivors as they view the concept of mental illness as a construct that

> is a part of the modernist project which devalues the diversity of human experience and perceptions and is preoccupied with analysis, eradication, physicality and mechanical and chemical constraint, rather than understanding, empathy, support and an holistic approach to the body and self.
>
> (Beresford and Wallcraft 1997: 71)

This antipathy towards what is, in effect, the legacy of Modernism and the Enlightenment is common to many contemporary social movements, but perhaps the user/survivor movement has most reason to be suspicious of its universalizing reason. After all, for Foucault (1967), it was the age of reason that gave us the modern conceptions of both madness and civilization. The influence of postmodernism can also be seen in the lack of a clear philosophy within the user/survivor movement. For example, while not without many internal critiques and debates, the social model of disability emerged as a clear philosophical position around which much of the physically disabled movement could cohere. However, while there are some within the user/survivor movement who have been influenced by the social model of disability because of its distinction between impairment and disability, others reject it on the basis that they do not view themselves as having an impairment nor as being disabled. This lack of a clear philosophy within the survivor movement does not concern some; on the contrary, it is seen as one of its strengths and attractions. Beresford and Wallcraft (1997) suggest this may be due to survivors' fears over substituting one rigid belief system, that of the medicalization of madness, with another which could, in a not dissimilar way, silence some of its members. Again the influence of postmodernism, summed up by Lyotard (1989: xxiv) as 'incredulity towards metanarratives', is evident in the way any Truth (with a capital T) is viewed with suspicion and is replaced by many truths, each claiming equal validity and the right to be heard.

Table 1 Self-identification and relationship to psychiatry

Type	Discourse	Orientation
Patient	'I am a schizophrenic'	Passive acceptance
Consumer	'I am a person with schizophrenia'	Compatible acceptance and resistance
Survivor	'I am a person who hears voices'	Active resistance

Source: Speed 2006: 29

This process of rejection of the categorization 'patient' and the consequent identification of an external source of oppression can be seen in the changing terminology of the movement. The earlier movements still identified themselves as 'mental patients', for example the Mental Patients Union (MPU) and Protection for the Rights of Mental Patients in Therapy (PROMPT). This began to change in the mid 1980s. PROMPT became the Campaign Against Psychiatric Oppression (CAPO) and newer organizations such as Survivors Speak Out and Mad Pride also rejected identification as a patient.

While somewhat simplistic, Speed's (2006) summary of the three typifications nevertheless helps illustrate the differences: see Table 1.

According to one activist, the 'term survivors was chosen to portray a positive image of people in distress and people whose experience differs from, or who dissent from, society's norms' (quoted in Barnes and Bowl 2001: 40). Survivors are people who seek to be seen as credible persons with rights of citizenship and who are therefore 'reluctant to enter or re-enter patienthood' (Pilgrim and Rogers 1999: 201). Such a position does not necessarily imply non-engagement with psychiatric services, though it would reject the reality of medical diagnoses; the emphasis is on active participation rather than passive patienthood or even negotiated consumerism, although the terms are not mutually exclusive and people can utilize a different discourse depending on the context of the speech act. It is being an active member of an organization resisting oppression that gives survivors their personal and political status. Speed, in what is the dominant view of the 'survivor discourse', sees it as arising 'out of a "claimed" rejection of the sick role (and a rejection of exclusion) and involves survivors portraying themselves as active agents' (Speed 2006: 30). In this view, survivor social movement organizations are seen as resisting psychiatric legitimacy, disputing its knowledge base and pursuing social and political change.

The politicizing process can be seen from analysing the discourse of survivors. Frequently, the language uses collective pronouns such as 'we' and 'us' rather than a more individualized identification. As Crossley and Crossley (2001) note:

> no longer are they purely individual experiences of a solitary ego. They are the experiences of a group; collective and shared experiences . . . [in addition] not only has the subject of experience been transformed. The object of experience has been transformed too. Injustices are no longer attributed to solitary doctors, institutions or nursing staff. Each individual case of mistreatment or injustice is now perceived and interpreted in terms of a generalized conception of 'the mental health system'. The generalized 'we' is oppressed by a collective 'them' or even an impersonal 'it'.
>
> (Crossley and Crossley 2001: 1484–1485)

It is also held that becoming an active 'survivor' rather than passive patient is empowering for the individual:

> Politicising oneself by joining with other survivors in political actions is an excellent antidote to the powerlessness that psychiatry induces in its subjects. Becoming active in the struggle against psychiatry (and other forms of injustice). . . is a good alternative to the helplessness psychiatry encourages.
>
> (Masson 1993: 319)

If the choice of language is a site of contestation, of power and resistance, it needs to be borne in mind that the decision to identify as survivor rather than as patient does not negate psychiatric power per se. In this sense, while the goal of 'empowerment' has become a key principle of modern day health and social policy, and while there has also been an erosion of the dominance of medical experts in terms of dictating care needs and treatment with an emphasis on negotiation, such is the dominance of the medical model and psychiatric profession that it is ultimately the doctors who hold the power. If they diagnose someone as suffering from a mental disorder, then under the existing law that is how they are categorized, and they can therefore find themselves subject to the full force of the psychiatric system.

Recognizing madness

People experiencing mental distress have been subject to various identities, many of which we would consider offensive today; from 'insane', 'loony' and 'mad' to 'schizo' and 'psycho', pejorative, value-laden and all-encompassing terms have served to label and stigmatize those on the receiving end. Terms such as 'mentally ill' have also been criticized for medicalizing social problems and objectifying the person, who, de facto, becomes the patient. The individual thus gets lost behind the diagnosis.

The domination of a powerful medical discourse not only constructs how the psychiatrist and patient relate to each other, but also allows the view of the former to be granted greater validity than that of the latter, with the patient often not being taken seriously at all. This can be seen in the way that intervention for physical ailments can be delayed as the symptoms are seen as due to mental problems, and personal liberty and autonomy can also be compromised by a diagnosis of mental illness.

This failure to acknowledge the patient's perspective, as we discussed above, has been criticized by many opponents of psychiatry. Not only is listening to what the patient says held to be crucial for professionals if they wish to understand and help their client, but also a failure to do so invalidates the patient's account and is said to add to their suffering. For Campbell (1992), psychiatry's failure to recognize and value his subjective experience has added to the damage he has suffered at its hands since the mid 1980s. This failure to recognize his experience, this *misrecognition*, is seen as intrinsically damaging.

The call therefore is for patients' voices to be heard, for them to be seen as experts in their own lives. This right to be heard, to have their voice accorded credibility, to have their experiences seen as valid and not subordinate to a medical Truth is one of the key demands of the user/survivor movement. The role of embodiment, of situated knowledge, is held to allow psychiatric survivor testimonials to become politicized challenges to mainstream biological reductionist psychiatry. As Canning (2006) argues,

> If embodied knowledge is to be acknowledged then those diagnosed as mentally ill must be viewed, at least in part, as experts of their own world, a world in which medical knowledge can only partly explain. An embodied, situated knowledge is about the telling of stories at a particular point in time from a particular – often oppressed – position. As healing and good mental health have been commodified, individualized, and characterized within the mind/body distinction, embodied knowledge, conversely,

challenges the political, economic, and social conditions in which one experiences mental illness *through the body*.

(Canning 2006, emphasis in original)

It should be clear then that the adoption of the psychiatric survivor identity is not akin to that of, for example, a cancer survivor. The latter individual has survived a physical disease; for the former the term is used to deny the very existence of disease and to denote unjust treatment and loss of liberty.

The call to listen to embodied experience does not necessarily preclude acknowledgement that scientific knowledge can explain certain aspects of human behaviour. Instead, it is more concerned with an overly deterministic aetiology and of how a focus on genetic or biological factors can preclude people diagnosed with schizophrenia from being seen as knowing their own world. The patient, who cannot know herself, is not a subject but an object of psychiatric knowledge, diagnosis and treatment. Listening to and validating the experiences of those in distress does not necessarily mean accepting the accounts as 100 per cent factually accurate. It does mean not silencing them as the unintelligible ramblings of the 'hysteric' or 'psychotic'.

Outside influences inside the head

The user/survivor movement is a historical phenomenon whose fields of possibilities have been both opened up and constrained by wider societal conditions. Such is the influence of external factors on movement development and individual and collective consciousness that Tomes' acknowledgement that in the USA 'the growing influence of consumer/survivor perspectives has largely been *a consequence, not a cause*, of radical restructurings of the mental health field' can equally be applied to the UK (Tomes 2006: 727, my emphasis).

So, while there are various courses of action that can be taken by individuals and groups at any given time, such opportunities can differ at specific historical moments due to various social and cultural forces. Most importantly in terms of the mental health movement is the closing down of the asylum system and the concomitant move to the hospital and community as the sites of care, control and contention. This change of field can enable certain forms of campaigning to open up while foreclosing others. For example, in the old long-stay hospitals, which were, in Goffman's (1961) term 'total institutions', strikes or the withholding of cooperation with the hospital authorities were forms of protest that could be utilized. However, being confined within the total institution away from wider society meant that other forms of protest, such as public petitions or demonstrations, were not possible (Crossley 2002b).

The wider cultural influences on how protest was articulated within the mental health movement are not difficult to see. The earlier movement, like many movements of the time, had a strong emphasis on social class and of working together with other oppressed groups, as can be seen by the Mental Patients Union statement contained in their 1972 'Fish Manifesto':

> Together with other oppressed groups, patients through an organized MENTAL PATIENTS UNION must take COLLEC-TIVE ACTION and realize their POWER in the CLASS STRUGGLE, alongside trade unions, Claimants Unions, Women's Liberation, Black Panther groups, Prisoner Rights etc.
> (quoted in Crossley 2002b: 54, emphasis in original)

Interviewees also reference the gay rights movement, the environmental movement and black activism. These activists identified with a more radical tradition of politics which influenced their worldview and the way in which they articulated strategies for change. Elements of class awareness and analysis still remain, for instance *Asylum*, the UK magazine, subtitled *The Magazine for Democratic Psychiatry*, published an editorial in 2002 revisiting the developments of the 1970s. The editorial was not only anti-medical but also located this within a class context, with the real struggle being seen as an 'ideological one, against the class nature of exclusion and for the decriminalization and depsychiatrization of irrationality and distress' (T. McLaughlin 2002: 3). The following year saw a special issue (vol. 13, no. 4), devoted to the late Pete Shaughnessy. Alongside his name and picture on the front cover are the words 'working class hero'. At the conference to mark the magazine's relaunch in 2009 (it had folded following the death of the editor Terence McLaughlin in September 2007), some speakers also addressed the issue of mental distress and alienation from a class-based viewpoint.

So, as in wider society, the issue of class remains the main focus for some. However, also reflective of wider society is the fact that the question of class, both in terms of consciousness and conflict, is no longer as dominant a framework through which political, societal and personal issues are discussed. It does not have anything like the same hold on working class consciousness today as it did up until the late

1970s and early 1980s. The articulation and attribution of alienation and mental distress takes different forms in the current period, although, interestingly, as we will discuss in the next chapter, as class and trade union activity recedes from the user/survivor movement, mental health issues have become a main focus of mainstream trade union activity, with unions increasingly presenting workplace conflict and the effects of capitalism in psychological terms, as being caused by such things as ' stress' and 'bullying' which require therapeutic support in response (Wainwright and Calnan 2002; Ecclestone and Hayes 2009).

Out of the bin and glad to be mad

The cultural turn in contemporary society has also influenced the survivor movement, and as class consciousness has diminished, the battle over cultural and lifestyle issues has risen. At the First National Conference of Survivor Workers UK, there was a strong emphasis on 'coming out' as a current or past psychiatric patient. The obvious influence here is from the gay and lesbian movement, where it took courage to be open about one's sexuality in a homophobic society. Similarly, the discrimination and hostility that can be aimed at users/survivors can also make people reluctant to admit to their experiences, to 'come out'. The survivor worker conference followed on from other developments whereby speaking openly about mental distress and/or psychotic experiences was encouraged. Mad Pride held its first event in 1999. Taking inspiration from the gay movement's reappropriation of erstwhile abusive terms such as 'queer' and the celebration of gay culture , 'mad activists' were also 'out and proud'. With the old asylums colloquially known as the 'bins', society's dustbins where those not wanted could be swept out of sight, the old gay pride slogan 'Out of the Closet and Glad to be Gay' could be modified and applied to Mad Pride activists, who were 'Out of the Bin and Glad to be Mad'.

Mad Pride festivals work on similar lines to Gay Pride events. Whereas gay activists celebrate gay identity and culture, mad activists celebrate mad identity and culture. Co-founded by Simon Barnett and Pete Shaughnessy, Mad Pride aimed to challenge negative perceptions of madness and to highlight the positives of 'mad culture'. It confronted society with the attitude that 'If you've got a problem with mad people, it's your problem' (Barnett 2008). A free festival held in the year 2000 attracted up to 4000 people according to the organization's co-founder.[3]

Here we see the influence of identity politics and the politics of recognition, the emphasis being on cultural aspects of life and the emotional and psychological effects of misrecognition rather than around the means of production or redistribution of wealth. This is not to say that financial considerations are ignored, and plans to oppose any reductions in welfare disability benefits by the Conservative/ Liberal Democrat coalition government were being formulated by Mad Pride in August 2010. Slogans to date include 'Bankers – Hands Off Our Welfare Benefits!'; 'Stop The Suicides – Hands Off Our Benefits!'; 'Back to Work? No Chance! Hands Off Our Benefits!' and 'Rich Scum! Hands Off Our Welfare Benefits!' (Mad Pride 2010).

From a pragmatic point of view, the campaign to protect welfare benefits is a laudable fight to protect the living standards and support needs of those in receipt of them. It does, however, highlight some of the tensions within identity politics and the demand to be recognized as 'mad'. The continuation of benefits entails the adoption of a medical framework in order for them to be accessed. It is ultimately the health and social care professionals who decide if the individual is 'mentally ill' enough to warrant payment or services. This runs the risk of reinforcing dominant paradigms at the same time as attempting to undermine them. It is also a telling sign of the times that the demand for the 'right to work' is heard less than that demanding the 'right to benefits'.

This also illustrates a further contradiction between identity politics based on class and that based on cultural recognition. As discussed in Chapter 2, the aim of working class activism was not to celebrate working class culture but to abolish class society, and with it itself as a class. The politics of recognition, on the other hand, seeks perpetuation and acknowledgement of said identity. Here, the goal is not to transcend but to accept identity. The more one is recognized positively as 'mad', the more one has to lose by rescinding that identity. This can be seen in the way that social policy around user/survivor involvement can give certain individuals increased social status in terms of self-esteem, respect, a certain amount of cultural or organizational power and perhaps even a salary. In such cases to lose the mad identity, to move *out* of the system can involve substantial loss. Recognition, as it is presented here, is not about a one-off acknowledgment of distress, on the contrary it is *constant recognition* that is required and in many cases demanded.

While much is progressive in the literature, art and practical solutions advanced by the user/survivor movement, the challenge ahead is how to distinguish the progressive from the regressive, and some of the positive and negative aspects of these developments have been discussed above. It is important to differentiate between individuals and groups who have experienced (or survived) the mental health system, and the institutionalization of 'surviving' whereby people are encouraged to identify themselves as such. This notion of continual recognition necessitates 'survivors' emphasizing and re-emphasizing their relationship with the psychiatric system, and those they interact with must duly recognize this relationship in a mutually re-enforcing dialogue that is past oriented. While many people encounter the psychiatric system during a period of crisis and despair, recover and get on with their lives, the survivor is imprisoned within the system in much the same way as the fixed identity of the asylum inmate. The imprisonment may not be physical, but in a psychological sense survivors are as trapped. To put their experiences behind them and get on with their lives necessitates foregoing the recognition received and losing their defining identity. The human ability to overcome adversity was compromised by the all embracing patient identity of the past. In challenging such a degrading view of humanity, the survivor movement needs to be careful that it does not discard the literal straitjacket for its metaphorical equivalent.

Conclusion

The rise of the psychiatric survivor has been influenced by many of the developments discussed in previous chapters. The declining significance of class politics and the move to a celebration of identity and culture is clearly discernible within the movement. Public and professional recognition of the validity of the subjective experience as being real for the individual is demanded, and the withholding of such recognition held to be further damaging to his or her sense of self.

Wider social change also played a key role, with the closing down of the asylums and the move to community care allowing a more public space for the articulation of distress and protest. If you were already confined in a long-stay institution, your ability to speak out publicly was obviously severely curtailed, and if you were in the community, awareness that the price of speaking out about your experiences and desires could see you incarcerated could prove an effective silencer.

In this respect both material and cultural changes in treatment and attitudes to madness have been crucial in the development of an active and vociferous psychiatric survivor movement. This articulation of trauma is paradoxical in that the disavowal of the status of patient in favour of a politically active survivor coexists with campaigns that emphasize vulnerability and dependence, as in demands for the right to claim sickness and incapacity benefits. This illustrates one danger of the embracing of an identity that keeps the activist confined within a system and discourse which they purport to reject.

Such a paradox, while highlighting the influence of the trauma-recognition-identity discourses on the survivor movement, is perhaps understandable, in that many of those in contact with the psychiatric services are in severe distress and/or disabled and in need of help and support. Often it is the nature of the 'support' offered and given that is contested, not the need for support per se.

Psychiatric survivors expressed concern with the medicalizing of the human condition and objectification of the person-as-patient that could result from this. Despite some success, just as in Chapter 3 we saw how the concept of trauma survivor expanded to include a growing number of people within its framework, in similar vein, psychiatric and psychological explanations are increasingly the prism through which social problems and the individual self are understood today. This development is the subject of the following chapter.

Notes

1 It should be noted that the diagnosis and treatment of physical ill health is itself not devoid of moral and political judgment (e.g. see Illich 1976).
2 His half-brother, Terry, had a diagnosis of schizophrenia. Terry killed himself in 1985.
3 While most activists are only too well aware of the reality and pain of severe mental distress, and seek to alleviate this for themselves and other people through a variety of means, it is still worth pointing out that there is a danger in the celebration of madness that the reality of the pain is undermined. This was tragically illustrated by the suicide of Pete Shaughnessy, co-founder of Mad Pride.

5   The rise of therapeutic identity

The demand for recognition is held by some to be the fundamental condition of human existence, the withholding of it deemed to be a negation of our humanity, misrecognition a mortal blow to our existence. However, as we have seen, the particular form that such demands take, what aspects of our existence that we want recognition for, is historically and culturally contingent, shaped by a complex interplay of socio-political factors and discursive practices, interwoven by power dynamics that influence our subjectivity and thus the articulated expression of our demand for recognition.

Increasingly in contemporary society, the form such demands take is through the prism of a therapeutic mode of understanding, of inherent vulnerability and the parallel notion of a self that is damaged and fragile. It is the recognition of past or present trauma that is demanded; recognition not in respect of what the individual or group has done but on what has been done to them, not for what they have achieved but what they have suffered. Increasingly, the political language used by such groups, and also by those politicians eager for their vote, is of demands that are made not on the grounds of universal citizenship, but to a special experience of suffering. Such articulation of a therapeutic narrative through which to understand experience is primarily presented as a caring, benign way to help people through a time of emotional pain. Helping people to cope with their difficulties in such a way is held to be empowering, a process through which they learn to deal with negative emotions, which in turn leads to an improvement in social functioning and independence. While it is the case that a professionally mediated narrative can have positive benefits, such as accessibility to medical and community resources and the provision of an explanation, however flawed, for the experience of emotional distress and/or exhibition of bizarre behaviour, there is a price to be paid for the adoption of such an account.

The complexity of a person's life, her social relations and the workings of power can be buried beneath the 'diagnosis', whether that is a formal psychiatric one or the location of the trauma to a specific past abusive event or relationship. To a greater or lesser extent, such diagnoses are concerned with causes not meanings, with traumatic *events*, specific *instances* rather than whole persons.

This chapter explores the trend whereby a therapeutic narrative has emerged as the dominant mode of expression for subjective distress and social dissatisfaction. Concomitant with this has been an expansion of psychological techniques and diagnostic criteria that has seen these disciplines move from the clinic to the wider social culture and in the process help shape our subjectivity.

Power and identity

Identification as a trauma survivor or psychiatric patient is accessible only via the incorporation of the self into expert discourses that are themselves instruments of power. In Foucauldian terms, such therapeutic explanations are 'truth effects', produced in discourse rather than being indicative of an objective entity that is the cause of subjective distress. Disciplines such as psychiatry, psychology and social work derive their power from their perceived ability to give us the 'real truth' about ourselves and the wider world. Knowledge and power are not two distinct spheres that operate independently, on the contrary they are intertwined; knowledge is produced in relation to power and is also influential of power.

Foucault's (1967, 1979, 1980) work was concerned with identifying the way in which 'practitioners of the soul' – psychiatrists, psychologists, social workers, therapists and counsellors – developed a panoply of powerful scientific and social techniques with which to categorize, treat and control individuals, for example in such things as the personality test, IQ test, psychiatric classifications, social work reports and risk assessments. In so doing, they do not simply describe the person but help to create them, not only as objects but also as subjects, due to the way in which they can also influence the individual's sense of self. We are embodied subjects; 'a subjectivity is produced in discourse as the self is subjected to discourse' (Parker 1989: 64).

The power of the psy-disciplines and other loci of power to construct a subject in a certain way also illustrates the illocutionary effect of language, whereby speech does not merely reflect reality but plays an active part in constructing it. When the psychiatrist utters the words, 'You are suffering from a mental illness; you have schizo-phrenia', in effect the recipient of such words finds that their status in society changes. As was discussed in Chapter 4, they are now the patient, the 'schizo', the mad, 'Other'. They can now be subject to mental health legislation that can see them detained in hospital and given medical treatment against their will, a power that now extends into the community with the introduction of community treatment orders in the Mental Health Act 2007, and which research shows is being used vigorously by risk-averse professionals to control their clients (McLaughlin 2010). In similar vein, the power of professionals to categorize the individual as, for example, asylum seeker, antisocial, at risk or a risk, plays a part in both actively constructing the subject and also allowing control to be exerted over them.

Foucualt's analysis of existing power/knowledge regimens was picked up by many looking for ways in which to develop oppositional strategies to dominant power relations. His critique of essentialist notions of identity influenced many radicals and has provoked intense debate (Sawicki 1991). Foucault's view that identity is a social, political and cultural issue rather than a given, fixed for all time, resonated within the feminist movement, unsurprisingly given feminist critiques of aspects of Enlightenment universalism and humanism as being used to justify women's oppression. However, Foucauldian analyses, insightful as many of them are, can downgrade the role of agency in the production of subjectivity. If our subjectivity is merely at the intersection of numerous power effects, then we are the product not the producer. As Benhabib (1992) puts it,

> If the subject who produces discourse is but the product of the discourse it has created. . . then the responsibility for this discourse cannot be attributed to the author but must be attributable to some fictive 'authorial position', constituted by the intersection of 'discursive planes'.
>
> (Benhabib 1992: 216)

The scope for social change is also reduced, the weight of power being seen as too great to be challenged by the mere 'objects' of history. Benhabib et al. (1995) see this problem of the degradation of agency in much poststructural thought, Butler's theory of performativity being criticized for being 'a doing without a doer' (Benhabib et al. 1995: 22). Foucault was aware of this danger in his work and did try to extricate himself from it by emphasizing that 'where there is power there is resistance' (Foucault 1979: 95), whereby certain discourses could be resisted and the subject could choose from a field of possibilities. Likewise, the idea that the discursively constituted subject lacks agency is rejected by feminists such as Sawicki (1991) and Butler (1990). For Butler (1990: 147), 'Construction is not opposed to agency; it is the necessary scene of agency', and she argues that her theory of performativity offers an account of how power and problematic binary divisions can be subverted. While such accounts do rescue a notion of human agency, this can be of a very limited nature, in that the constant reiteration of performance can reduce the speed of change to mere evolutionary pace. This also ignores the radical ruptures of social change that have been experienced on occasions during the past three centuries (Heartfield 2002).

While Foucault's work is not without problems it has been hugely influential as many writers try to incorporate and develop his insights. The political context and consequent social relations in which discursive practices are established was emphasized by many (e.g. Parker 1989). Wetherell and Potter (1992) distinguish between 'constitutive discourse' and 'established discourse'. This acknowledges that subjects are both *constituted* within discourse but also that said discourse has not arisen from nowhere but has been *established* through human agency, albeit under particular social conditions.

In this sense the task is to view the processes through which a certain construction of the subject is established, which entails the deconstruction of the subject, which, for Derrida, is among other things, 'the genealogical analysis of the trajectory through which the concept of the subject has been built, used and legitimised' (quoted in Walia 2004, online).

A useful way of conceptualizing the emergence of the subject from its surroundings is that of the 'triple helix self', by which Wainwright and Calnan (2002) seek to extend Marx's observation that 'Men make their own history, but they do not make it just as they please; they do not make it under circumstances chosen by themselves, but under circumstances directly encountered, given and transmuted from the past (Marx 1978 [1852]: 595). In the triple helix self, the three strands of the helix represent the natural environment, discourse and corporeality respectively. As Wainwright and Calnan (2002) point out,

> Mind or subjectivity emerges from the helix as the three points spiral around each other across the life course. As well as illustrating the formation of the self at a particular point in time (the head of the helix), the model also reveals the biographical-historical dimensions of the self (the tail of the helix), as

historically specific environmental conditions and discursive formations interact with corporeality across time. It is important to
recognize that the tail of the helix predates the birth of the individual because corporeality (in the form of genetic material), and
obviously discourse and the external environment, already exist
(and already interact) before the emergence of the individual self.

(Wainwright and Calnan 2002: 85–86)

In this sense it is important to understand why, in the contemporary
period, the interaction of the three strands of the helix leads to the
formation of the self as sick and traumatized, while more and more
social interactions are viewed through a psychological prism. The
widespread adoption of a therapeutic sensibility within wider society
is marked by an increased sense of societal anxiety, individual vulnerability and estrangement – from each other, traditional forms of
authority and political institutions. One outcome of the many complex dynamics affecting contemporary subjectivity is that therapeutic
categorizations and ways of thinking are no longer confined to the
clinic or formal therapeutic encounter between analyst and analysand,
but have permeated popular culture, most notably in western societies
(Nolan 1998; Ecclestone and Hayes 2009).

From clinic to culture

The expansion of psychiatric and psychological theories and disciplinary techniques has been well documented and criticized from
both within (e.g. Szasz 1961; Parker et al. 1995; Thomas 1997) and
outwith the psy-disciplines (e.g. Reiff 1966; Nolan 1998; Furedi 2004).
Indeed, the influence of the psy-complex can be traced back to the late
nineteenth and early twentieth centuries, with competing theories and
critiques offered as to both the positive and negative consequences of
such a way of understanding both the individual and collective
psyche. Likewise, the tendency to pathologize a range of 'problem'
behaviours and to use broad indicators to allow more people to fall
within such classifications is not a particularly novel development.
The Child Guidance movement, formed in Britain after the First
World War to work with 'maladapted' children, included such characteristics as 'shyness' and 'reserve' as aspects of maladaptation. In
addition, vigilance was required over ostensibly healthy children as
they were considered potentially susceptible to mental illness (Stewart
2009). Other disciplines, such as social work, also embraced elements
of psychological approaches, especially in relation to child develop-

ment and psychiatric social work. While the exact influence of psychoanalytic and other psychological theories within social work practice is disputed (Bree 1970), they had enough influence for some to question whether such employees were primarily social workers or therapists (Irvine 1978), and others to argue that social workers were being trained in a manner that precluded any political understanding of their work (Jordan and Parton 1983).

The 1980s and 1990s saw a continual expansion of therapeutic initiatives within the broader UK culture such that by the early 1990s counselling was firmly established in general medical practice (Pringle and Laverty 1993), with half of surgeries employing one by the end of the decade (Eatock 2000). Such a development is necessary, we are told, due to the poor mental health of the population. The Mental Health Foundation (MHF 1999) published a report claiming that 20 per cent of the UK's children were suffering from a mental health problem. Such a figure was an underestimate according to one psychiatrist giving evidence to a parliamentary committee, who suggested that the true figure was around 40 per cent (Marin 1996). Neither are such problems confined to children: one media-friendly psychologist is of the opinion that one-third of Britain's adult population exhibits signs of psychiatric morbidity (James 1997).

This process of psychologization was not confined to the clinic or surgery but began to filter through the mainstream media and popular discourse. Furedi (2004) cites research on UK newspapers that charted the rise in usage of such terms as self-esteem (no citations in 1980, 3 in 1986 103 in 1990 to 3328 in 2000); trauma (from under 500 citations in 1994 to over 5000 in 2000); stress (from under 500 in 1993 to just under 24,000 in 2000); syndrome (from under 500 in 1993 to over 6500 in 2000) and counselling (from under 500 in 1993 to over 7000 in 2000). This is a quite remarkable expansion in such a short period of time and provides compelling evidence that the language of therapy has now permeated broader culture. It is not that the problems facing us have changed significantly; people still live in poverty, suffer relationship problems and/or breakdown, worry over exam results, lose their jobs, have conflict in the workplace, suffer bereavements and experience existential angst. However, how we articulate these problems and how they are presented to us in contemporary discourse would appear to have undergone a remarkable transformation in the latter decades of the twentieth century.

Into the twenty-first century and the situation does not appear to have improved. In the USA a psychiatrist claims that one in ten nursery children are mentally ill (McLaughlin 2005), while in the UK mental health charities such as Mind routinely claim that 25 per cent of us are currently suffering, or will suffer from at a future point, a mental health problem. A wide range of popular and specialist therapeutic techniques are now firmly embedded in the education curriculum, whether at nursery, primary or high school, and also within the university system (Ecclestone and Hayes 2009). The UK government is reportedly committed to measuring the subjective well-being of the population, including an index to measure 'happiness' (*Guardian* 15 November 2010). No doubt further therapeutic interventions will follow for those who fail to reach the required level of psychological contentment.

The psychologization of social and political life also illustrates the blurring of what constitutes the left and right of politics today. For instance, the tendency to use psychological terminology is not confined to those of a conservative nature seeking simple explanations for the complexity of human subjectivity. On the contrary, to criticize the therapeutic turn can lead to accusations of being a right winger unsympathetic to the psychological suffering of the distressed. Also, those who consider themselves left wing are not averse to using the language of psychology against their opponents; terms such as homophobia and 'Islamophobia' are often used to describe those who harbour a dislike or prejudice towards homosexuals or those who follow the Islamic religion. The implication is that such an attitude is 'irrational' which can overlook the historical, ideological, political and social factors in which such attitudes develop.

The tendency to portray your political opponents as mentally ill is not new. It is well known, and been roundly condemned, that in the former Soviet Union psychiatrists often classified the regime's political opponents as suffering from mental disorder. In effect, dissent was pathologized; failure to follow the political orthodoxy ran the risk of psychiatric diagnosis and incarceration. However, such a move is not confined to erstwhile Stalinists. In similar vein, some environmental campaigners seek to label their opponents as mentally irrational, suggesting that climate change deniers or sceptics are suffering from a psychological illness. For example, in March 2009 the University of the West of England (UWE) at Bristol held a conference on the psychology of climate change denial. The news release advertising the conference opens with the axiomatic statement: 'Man-made climate change poses an unprecedented threat to the global ecosystem', and that the conference will consider the possibility that those not subscribing to this view are suffering from an 'addiction to consumption' (UWE 2009, online).

So, when claims are made that contemporary culture is dominated by psychologization, in which social and existential problems are increasingly viewed through a therapeutic prism, it could be argued that we are merely witnessing the continuation of a trend that was evident to some observers during the early twentieth century and to many during the latter decades of that century. It is certainly the case that there is no clean break between the past and the present, no precise date or event that in and of itself marks contemporary psychologization from its earlier versions. Nevertheless, we can delineate some changes which, in interaction with other dynamics, mark the present period from the past.

The rise of big pharma and the psychology industry

There have been various attempts to explain the therapeutic turn in contemporary society. Dineen (1999) likens what she terms the 'psychology industry' to any other industry in a capitalist economy. In order to survive, it must expand and open up new markets. In this process new problems and 'disorders' are created that necessitate the intervention of the therapeutic professional. From this perspective it is not the demand for therapy that creates the supply of therapists, but the opposite process; the supply of therapists creates the demand for therapy. This is a similar argument to that used by those who implicate the pharmaceutical industry for the rise in prescription medication. Rather than psychiatric medication being developed to treat an existing illness, in many cases the development of the pill precedes the identification of that which it is then said to treat and/or cure; the use of selective serotonin reuptake inhibitors (SSRIs) for 'social anxiety disorder' or 'night eating syndrome' and Viagra for 'sexual dysfunction' are some recent examples of where the pill existed long before the discovery of the 'illness' for which it is now prescribed (Lane 2007; Goldacre 2009). The drug companies are certainly powerful players in this, spending substantial amounts of money on the creation and promotion of their wares to treat an ever expanding number of mental 'disorders'. They take great care to ingratiate themselves with psychiatric professionals and are also substantial sources of revenue for the medical journals in which they frequently advertise their products. In subtle ways they blur the boundary between severe mental distress and everyday stresses and strains. For example, an advert in the *British Journal of Psychiatry* in October 1997 for the antidepressant Seroxat informs us that the drug 'helps get depressed patients back to normal, liberating them from everyday stresses and anxiety'. In such a way drug companies, via a hospitable medical medium, promote the pathologization of everyday life.

In similar vein there are many who blame psychiatric professionals for the exponential expansion of clinical diagnostic criteria. For example, between the first and fourth editions of the American Psychiatric Association's *Diagnostic and Statistical Manual*, published in 1952 and 1994 respectively, the number of pages grew from 130 to 886 and the number of diagnostic categories more than tripled. This led some sceptics to suggest, tongue only slightly in cheek, that at such a rate of growth we can reasonably expect the fifth edition to contain some 1256 pages and 1800 diagnostic criteria (Blashfield and Fuller 1996). The inclusion of diagnostic categories in the DSM is far from an objective, scientific process; on the contrary it can be driven by external and internal political concerns and deals, as well as by petty personal disagreements. In his illuminating account of such internal machinations during the writing of DSM-III, Lane (2007) notes the often bitter infighting between many of the psychiatrists involved in the process of approving diagnoses for inclusion in the manual, noting the irony that such hostility emanated from those charged with setting the benchmark for sociable interaction. He charts the process leading to the inclusion of *social phobia* as a psychiatric disorder in DSM-III in 1980 and also the way in which slight changes in terminology allowed the 'disorder' to apply to a greatly increased number of the population when the DSM-III revised edition (APA 1987) was published in 1987:

> While DSM-III had defined social phobia as 'a persistent, *irrational* fear of, and compelling desire to avoid, situations in which [we're] exposed to scrutiny by others', seven years later the description had morphed into 'a persistent fear of *one* or more situations (the social phobic situations) in which the person is exposed to *possible* scrutiny by others *and fears that he or she may do something or act in a way that will be humiliating or embarrass-ing*'. By silently deleting the proviso that these fears be 'irrational' and multiple, the second task force made the diagnosis so mild and causal that it could actually include, as an example of 'social phobic situations', a fear of sounding foolish.
>
> (Lane 2007: 100, emphasis in original)

A similar rhetorical process occurred in the production of the eighth edition of the European manual the *International Classification of*

Diseases (ICD-8: World Health Organization 1965). Previous editions included phrases such as 'schizophrenic reaction' or 'anxious reaction', but these became exclusively referred to as schizophrenia and anxiety. The verb became a noun, the person a diagnosis. Rather than having a reaction, whether of a schizophrenic or anxious type, you now had schizophrenia or anxiety. These developments were also incorporated into DSM-III. With DSM-V due to be published in 2012 we will have to wait before finding out the exact contents. However, early evidence suggests that the trend to categorize more behaviours within its pages will continue, with reports suggesting tortured discussions among those preparing it as to whether such things as overuse of the internet, 'excessive' sexual activity, compulsive shopping and apathy should be contained within the parameters of clinically diagnosable mental disorders in the next edition of the manual (Lane 2009). There has been some debate in wider society about the validity and/or expansion of the concept of post-traumatic stress disorder. For instance a 2009 BBC *Panorama* programme detailed the expansion of the concept from extreme experiences (for example, war situations) to the more mundane (for example, minor traffic accidents, work stress). At the end of that edition of *Panorama*, presenter Jeremy Vine said the APA was looking at tightening up the diagnostic criteria for PTSD in DSM-V. Time will tell if he is correct, but he is obviously unaware of posttraumatic embitterment disorder (PTED), an 'illness' said to afflict those who remain bitter or aggrieved for too long about a past wrong, and which some psychiatric professionals wish to be included in the new manual (Linden 2003).

Materialist influences

A more materialist analysis is given by Cloud (1998), who claims the rise of the therapeutic to be 'a political strategy of contemporary capitalism, by which dissent is contained within a discourse of individual or family responsibility' (Cloud 1998: xiii). Such an analysis could be extended to the problematizing of certain behaviours. For example, the focus on shyness, or 'social phobia' or 'avoidant personality disorder' could be seen as pathologizing those who fail to live up to the go-getting, gregarious entrepreneur of an individualist free market economy. Likewise, a desire for 'quick fix' solutions to the problems of life and concomitant wish to avoid complex social, political and existential issues by attributing all unpleasant emotional responses to faulty neurotransmitters, would favour the maintenance of the status quo rather than that of radical change.

Despite coming from a Marxist standpoint, Cloud (1998) nevertheless sees collusion on the part of some Marxist and feminist thinkers and activists in this process due to their advocating a 'politics of self-expression', a 'revolution from within'. This focus on the immediate terrain of individual consciousness is held to be the necessary starting point with which individual suffering can be put into some form of social understanding and political action. In this sense, the early feminist focus on the body, self-help and analysis was because they saw it as a legitimate site for intervention in the pursuit of wider political action.

Gradually, however, there was a change of focus. Haaken discusses this in relation to the sexual abuse movement, and notes how there was a profound shift during the 1980s whereby it became 'more centred on demonstrating the damage inflicted on women than asserting their intactness' (Haaken 1998: 86). She also suggests that the focus on past sexual abuse may be influenced by gendered power dynamics in the present: 'As some women achieve subjective authority within public life and yet find themselves continuing to be subjugated by powerful men, it may be less dangerous to confront the "dead" fathers of early childhood than the living ones' (Haaken 1998: 93). Similarly, the focus on the church as a site of widespread child abuse may be partly explained due to it being easier to generate unity of moral outrage over the priest's sexual abuse of a child than the church's pronouncements on homosexuality, abortion or the role of women in society.

Haaken is certainly not implying that sexual abuse does not happen or is not traumatic, but rather, is acknowledging that all narrative accounts contain multiple levels of meaning and are mediated via complex social, cultural, political and power dynamics; 'the pasts that are recovered in individual or collective remembering are transformed by the dilemmas of the present' (Haaken 1998: 275). For example, she argues that

> Throughout the 1980s, the decline of an activist women's movement and the rise of political conservatism took a heavy toll on grassroots organizations. Political programs targeting sexual abuse of children survived while other programs, including domestic-battering and poverty related services, did not because sexuality was the one area where feminists could enlist conservative support and moral outrage.
>
> (Haaken 1998: 241)

If the role of religious power and influence is significant in relation to the focus on the issue of sexual abuse, some argue that it is the relative decline of religion as a cohering force in the contemporary period that has influenced the growth of a therapeutic culture (e.g. Hunter 2000). As society becomes more secular, there are many who see the rise of the therapist/counsellor as the replacement for the priest or imam. Instead of going to see the priest for guidance on how to lead our lives in such a way as to achieve 'salvation', we instead visit the therapist for 'life coaching' to allow us to achieve salvation's contemporary equivalent, 'good mental health'. However, again it would be a mistake to see the decline of religion and rise of the therapeutic as cause and effect. As Furedi (2004) points out,

> In the past the 'death of God' was not linked to the valorisation of emotion, but to the growing significance attached to science and reason. In the twentieth century, the rise of the new ideologies of communism, socialism and fascism were represented as meeting the need created by the death of religion.
>
> (Furedi 2004: 91)

As people attempt to give their lives meaning, to make sense of their experiences, it does seem plausible that as the old sources of authority lose their ability to play such a role then other players will come forward to fill the vacuum. Lasch was also concerned with the loss of cultural authority, particularly in the USA, although his focus was on the decline of parental authority from the mid-nineteenth century onwards. He noted how 'schools, peer groups, mass media and the "helping professions" had challenged parental authority and taken over many of the family's child-rearing functions', a process that influenced a 'culture of narcissism' (Lasch 1991: 238).

While a critical analysis of the role of 'Big Pharma', the psychology industry, and the workings of those responsible for compiling the 'official' list of 'mental disorders' do provide us with many insights, there is, however, a tendency to reify such players and institutions, attributing to them omniscient powers with which they beguile a passive population. Neither individual psychologists, nor an all powerful psychology or pharmaceutical industry, can account for the above trends. They are certainly influential players, but people are not mere objects into which professional explanations and treatments can simply be poured. Likewise, the identification of social changes is important, but again, no one change in isolation can account for the widespread acceptance of a therapeutic sensibility. Instead, a much more complex social and cultural dynamic is at play.

It was this to which Szasz (1991) was referring when he argues that the classification of people into diagnostic categories requires three different types of persons: the classifier (doctor/therapist), classified (patient) and, importantly, 'a public called upon to accept or reject a particular classification' (Szasz 1991: 53). At various times we play all three roles; we classify people, we are classified and we are members of a society in which some classifications are viewed more positively than others. However, as Szasz (1991) points out, we can accept or reject this process. The issue then is if such explanations are more accepted today than in the past, then what is it about contemporary society that has allowed such ideas to gain such a strong foothold in society? Is it possible, as many of the writers cited above suggest, to isolate one particular variable above all others, whether feminism, religion or the family, as the most important factor in the rise of the therapeutic ethos? These are the questions addressed in detail by Nolan (1998) in the USA and Furedi (2004) in the UK, both of whom argue that we are witnessing a redrawing of the relationship between the state and the individual, particularly as old sources of moral authority are increasingly seen as discredited or irrelevant to present day circumstances. The strength in their work is the focus on the complex interplay between cultural and political change in the shaping of individual and collective subjectivity.

The transformation of the sick role

One cultural change has been a transformation of the sick role. To be ill or sick nowadays does not necessarily imply the negation of the self. There has been a move from a cultural outlook that accorded 'positive valuation of health and the negative valuation of illness between therapeutic agent and sick persons' (Parsons 1978: 76), to one where the dividing line between health and illness, disabled and non-disabled, sanity and insanity is hotly contested. Disability, whether mental or physical, is held to be a social construction, and people with a disability become 'Other' to the non-disabled gaze, objects for investigation, treatment and control due to the knowledge/ power nexus. In some instances, the 'positive' aspects of illness, disability or madness are emphasized. As discussed earlier, the Mad Pride organization, among others, celebrates the positive aspects of madness. Many within the Deaf community see themselves not as having a disability but as a linguistic and cultural minority. Such aspects of their identity are accorded positive, not negative, status. From this perspective, it is the continuation of that particular trait, not its eradication by way of a 'cure' that is embraced. As such it can then become a defining part of individual and group identity, and consequently the search for a cure for deafness can be seen as akin to genocide, the extermination of a devalued minority.

With the dividing lines blurred and the positive aspects of disability proclaimed, it should be little surprise if there is at times a demand for a diagnosis. In such circumstances, to refuse to diagnose, or to question the validity of a diagnosis can court hostility. This marks a change from the anti-psychiatry arguments of the 1960s and 1970s where diagnoses were deconstructed and ridiculed by psychiatry's critics. The changing cultural climate was highlighted by the differing reception for two books by the American literary critic and feminist, Elaine Showalter, *The Female Malady* (1985) and *Hystories: Hysterical Epidemics and Modern Culture* (1997). While the first book enjoyed much acclaim and is deemed essential reading for any serious student of the relationship between gender and mental health, the later one provoked much criticism, with Showalter having to encounter public protests at several post-publication promotional events.

The difference was not so much in what she was arguing, but in the cultural environment in which it was expressed. In many respects, Showalter was making the same point in both books; that what are often termed medical diseases or illnesses are actually the result of complex social, political and psychological processes that could get hidden under a psychiatric diagnosis. However, the later book was published in a climate far less amenable to deep searches for meaning in human experience. Instead, catch-all simple diagnoses and professional expertise, whether by way of therapy or medication, are now seen as holding the key to the understanding of human suffering.

In such a climate, to question someone's diagnosis can be taken as an attack on their integrity, as a failure to confer on them due recognition. As was discussed in Chapter 2, the withholding of recognition is held to be a grievous blow to someone's sense of identity, the infliction of a grievous psychological scar. However, such political campaigns to have the victim's voice heard and legitimized can lead to a cul-de-sac where it is not considered acceptable to bring in factors from the wider social world that have played a part in the cultivation of such an identity.

Of course, there are many who will use their diagnosis for financial reasons. Claims for compensation frequently rely on the pathologization of emotion and experience. For example, PTSD is now a common component in compensation cases in Britain, with even employees of the army, navy, police and ambulance services suing on the grounds of trauma suffered during the course of their work. Medical insurance claims also require a diagnosis, as Kirk and Kutchins (1997) point out:

Now, mental health professionals must label their clients as pathological in order for them to be reimbursed by their insurance companies. Suddenly a woman seeking help in coping with an unpleasant boss is defined as clinically depressed; or a housewife who voices concern about her shopping sprees is labelled bi-polar (manic depressive).

(Kirk and Kutchins 1997: cover)

Kirk and Kutchins (1997) were primarily concerned with developments in the USA but the popularization of PTSD soon crossed the Atlantic to the UK. Firefighters who attended the football stadium fire in Bradford in 1985 and those present at the Kings Cross underground fire in 1987 claimed compensation due to resultant PTSD, as did many police officers and fans at the Hillsborough football stadium disaster in 1989.

In relation to claims by those police officers at Hillsborough, one High Court judge tried to insist that police officers 'will not be persons of ordinary phlegm, but of extraordinary phlegm hardened to events which would to ordinary persons cause distress' (House of Lords 1998). Such a rearguard action in defence of resilience contrasts with that of those psychologists who claim that the prevalence of PTSD in police officers may be as much as six times higher than for the general population, affecting up to 18 per cent of the constabulary. A similar percentage of firefighters are also said to be affected by symptoms of PTSD (Green 2004). When you consider that the diagnosis became formally recognized by the American Psychiatric Association only in 1980, its absorption into the wider social world has taken place at breakneck speed. The trauma survivor is no longer in the minority; on the contrary such an identification is now increasingly commonplace.

Conclusion

Heightened anxiety in society at the loss of older sources of authority, particularly when new ones have yet to appear and/or gain widespread acceptance, can leave people more susceptible to individualistic, psychological interpretations of life problems. However, such events are not directly causal. Concerns over the death or decline of religion have been around for the past two centuries without a corresponding embrace of therapy culture. In other words a turn towards the therapeutic is not the inevitable outcome of a secular society. Likewise, concern over the decline of parental authority or the role of the family is not particularly new, so, on their own, cannot account for the embracement of psychological explanations for contemporary social and existential problems. Neither the pharmaceutical companies nor psychology industry are able to exercise the control over society that their critics suggest, their success has less to do with their power than with a broader political and cultural climate in which their messages are mediated.

Therefore, while each may be a significant factor, on their own they do not provide us with a sufficient explanation for the contemporary zeitgeist. In addition, the present epoch is one in which science and reason no longer command such exalted status. As discussed in earlier chapters, science is often portrayed as a destructive threat to humanity and the planet, while reason stands accused of being a chimera, a means by which the powerful subjugate the powerless, and the twentieth century political ideologies have lost their significance. The rise of the therapeutic then is linked to complex social dynamics and political change. To expand on this further, I wish to look at the influence of some further political developments in the cultivation of the psychologically vulnerable subject.

6   The imposition of a vulnerable identity

Present day society is no longer primarily concerned with attaining something good but with preventing the worst. This anticipation of something going wrong at a later date informs action in the present and is what Beck (1992: 33) refers to as the 'Not-Yet-Event as stimulus for action'. From such a perspective the individual is seen as one who is at risk, as more object than subject, increasingly powerless in the face of omniscient and omnipresent malevolent forces. This symptom of cultural and indeed political malaise in western society was highlighted by Sontag (1989) in relation to the panic about AIDS in the late 1980s. She perceptively noted 'the striking readiness of so many to envisage the most far-reaching of catastrophe' (Sontag 1989: 4), and that rather than a case of 'Apocalypse Now' there was a sense of 'Apocalypse from now on'.

If the population is more anxious and susceptible to therapeutic explanations for the problems of life today, then another factor to consider is the extent to which the politics of fear have played in the creation of such a situation. Indeed, it is remarkable how many opposing political traditions and social groupings share a common tactic of propagating fear and anxiety in the population. The neo-cons in London and Washington highlight the danger from such things as fundamentalist terror attacks and 'rogue' states, the remnants of the left and new environmentalist groups highlight the danger of such things as climate change, global warming and genetically modified crops.

According to Clare Short, former cabinet minister in the Labour government, 'Very soon, human civilisation will collapse and human life become unliveable' (Short 2009: 65). While few would consider Short on the radical wing of progressive politics, her claim resonates with the wider proclamations from those who do claim the radical mantle. Campaign groups of various hues warn us of the dangers of domestic violence, child abuse, predatory paedophiles, bird flu, swine flu, bullying, AIDS and other sexually transmitted diseases, our sedentary or hectic lifestyles, stress, and numerous threats to our well-being from the food we eat, to name but a few. Trade unions frequently warn us of the threats we face from 'bullying' or 'stress inducing' managers and colleagues (McLaughlin 2008). A walk around any university campus in the UK will find an array of posters warning students of the potential dangers facing them on and off campus. University life, once a time of engagement with ideas, of intellectual stimulation, the first step towards adult independence away from the parental gaze, of making mistakes but learning from them, could now be reasonably perceived by students as a place where if not their life, then certainly their health was at serious risk. Today, a dominant political slogan could be said to be 'Left and Right, Unite and Fright'.

Wider political change has led to the coalescence of virtually all political groupings around the threat of looming catastrophe whether on an individual or global scale. In these readings we are all assumed to be vulnerable due to our powerlessness and/or lack of awareness of the dangers we face. The expansion of the concept of vulnerability can be further illustrated by looking at the way it has become institutionalized within social policy. As discussed earlier, the concept of trauma is now the prism through which much grievance is expressed, with many social movements, individuals and campaign groups demanding that such trauma be afforded public affirmation and recognition. The assumption is that vulnerability is a normal condition for people to be in and that they require the input of a professional to allow them to regain control over their lives. If the role of many psy-professionals in promoting their wares has been well documented, relatively little has been said about the way the term 'vulnerability' has become institutionalized within politics and social policy. In the process, more and more people become officially vulnerable and in need of protection, which necessitates further state intervention into the affairs of the population. This psychologization of society, for all the rhetoric about empowerment, the alleviation of trauma and distress, and the ability for individual growth, actually represents a diminished view of the human potential.

This chapter illustrates this by looking at areas of work and social interaction that have in recent years been recast as toxic environments containing numerous threats to people's well-being. It also provides concrete examples from social policy that while often presented as benign measures to help and protect people, have been influenced by many of the factors discussed in previous chapters, and which contain paternalistic and authoritarian consequences.

United in stress: the role of the trade unions

The subject of stress, and in particular work-related stress, is illustrative of the way in which an aspect of subject identification is influenced by societal changes. The exposure to the harmful effects of stress is said to start at a young age. At its 1999 annual conference the Professional Association of Teachers denounced school examinations due to the pressure and resultant stress they put on students (*The Times* 28 July 1999). Exposure to 'stress' is said to be more harmful than exposure to violence (Thompson 1999). Stress is frequently cited as the cause of much personal pain and is said to be damaging to the economy in terms of stress-related absences by staff (Cooper and Cartwright 1994), and is also a burden on medical services as they attempt to contain and cure this apparent medical phenomenon. Such is its apparent ubiquity today, that it requires noting that 'stress' is actually a relatively recent historical construction. The word did not appear in the *Penguin Dictionary of Psychology* in 1952, nor in reprints up to 1963. Neither did the word 'counselling', one of the favoured treatments for 'stress'.

One reason for the label of stress being used to explain more and more experiences and emotions is that the term lacks clear definition. As Patmore (2006) notes, it can be both cause and effect, interaction and transaction, verb and noun. For example, caring for a sick or disabled relative is said to expose one to stress, which leads one to suffer stress. Exposure to stress is said to cause stress. In other words, stress causes itself. Despite, or perhaps because of this lack of clarity, increasingly, workplace relations between employer and employee, and also tensions between employees are being mediated by the trade unions and understood through a discourse of stress.

In April 2010 a general election was announced. The preceding weeks had seen British Airways cabin crew go on strike in a dispute over staffing cuts. Their union, Unite, is a major donor to the Labour party. Rail workers were also planning strike action during the same period. Perhaps inevitably, the Conservatives took this opportunity to argue that New Labour is really old Labour in disguise, in hock to the unions, still socialist at heart, and given the chance will return us to the 'dark days' of the industrial unrest of the 1970s and 1980s.

Such posturing betrays a lack of understanding of the extent to which things have changed. The Labour and Conservative parties of today bear little relation to their previous incarnations, having shed their old ideological positions and their connection to previous constituencies; the working class and trade union movement for Labour, the ruling class for the Conservatives. In terms of industrial action, the aforementioned strikes stand out only because of their rarity, and are far removed from the large scale and often brutal clashes of yesteryear such as the Winter of Discontent of 1978–79 or the year-long miners' strike of 1984–85. Approximately 29 million working days were lost in 1979, a mere 455,000 days in the whole of 2009 (Hume 2010).

Nowadays, the unions are more likely to portray their members as vulnerable individuals rather than as a collective body of strength. Instead of encouraging the workforce to take industrial action by going on strike, they are more likely to encourage workers to take industrial *inaction* by going off sick, and to then chaperone them through the courts in pursuit of a claim for compensation (Patmore 2006). Industrial relations, which previously focused on workers' rights, pay and conditions, are increasingly concerned with workers' emotions, and these are frequently articulated through the discourse of stress, with rest and counselling portrayed as the solution. For Patmore (2006), this 'best to rest' ethos represents the new opiate of the masses.

A number of factors are at play in the changing role of the trade union movement in how they frame and negotiate workplace conflict. From a political perspective, the decline of the trade union movement is intertwined with the decline of the working class as a political force in British politics, the defeat of the wider Left and loss of ideological coherence, perhaps most graphically symbolized by the tearing down of the Berlin Wall in 1989.

The origins of such a process long predate 1989, but the defeats of the 1980s acted as a catalyst for its acceleration. In a detailed account of the rise of the phenomenon of 'work stress', Wainwright and Calnan (2002) regard the defeat of the miners' strike of 1984–85 as a pivotal moment. This was a defeat which effectively marked the end of the working class as a major collective political force in the country. They note how, as the dispute wore on and victory looked less likely, the miners' signs, slogans and representations changed:

> At the beginning of the dispute the miners were confident of winning: placards and badges made assertive militant demands: 'Coal not Dole', 'Victory to the miners'. But by the time of their eventual defeat the mood and the slogans had changed: 'Dig deep

for the miners', 'Don't let them starve'. Rather than the image of the self-confident, politically conscious rank and file militant, the striking miners had become victims and charity cases.

(Wainwright and Calnan 2002: 140)

This is not to criticize the miners, who throughout the dispute faced the full force of the capitalist state (police brutality, media bias, withholding of benefits, etc.) with tremendous courage and resistance. However, for many reasons it soon became clear that the prospect of success seemed remote. In the process, a once strong and collective body was recast as vulnerable victims in need of protection. Following this defeat there was a refocusing by trade unions on the way in which they articulated workplace conflict, increasingly representing the individual rather than the collective worker, with a focus on issues of health and safety at work. However, this came at a price; the adoption of a therapeutic discourse in which workplace conflict was recast as a health issue, and the rise of the discourse of stress was a key outcome of this. In the process the individual worker was reduced to a passive object at the mercy of a toxic environment that was hazardous to his or her health, often due to 'bullying' by management or colleagues (McLaughlin 2008).

The rise of the term bullying, once almost exclusively confined to the school playground is indicative of the psychologization of the workplace and the attribution of vulnerability to employees. 'Workplace bullying' is now seen as a major threat to the health of Britain's workforce. Whether it is peer bullying or bullying by management towards staff, there is a growing consensus that there is a significant problem. The Trades Union Congress (TUC) declared 7 November 2007 as 'National Ban Bullying at Work Day'. Such is the apparent scale of the problem that some argue – without a hint of embarrassment – that workplace bullying is 'the second greatest social evil after child abuse' (Field 1996).

The Universities and College Union (UCU) has distributed posters which are displayed around campus informing us that 'Bullies Are a Workplace Hazard'. Staff common rooms have posters warning that there is 'No Entry for Bullies'. No doubt such posters are displayed with the best of intentions. However, by equating problems in the school playground with those in the workplace, they infantilize the workforce and view its vulnerability as axiomatic.

The Trades Union Congress established a 'Commission on Vulnerable Employment' that defined 'workers in vulnerable employment' as those experiencing poverty and injustice resulting from 'an imbalance of power in the employer-worker relationship' (TUC 2008: 3). The employer–worker power imbalance is not a new development. What is relatively recent is the way the workforce are considered weak, at risk and in need of help. Increasingly, as Ecclestone and Hayes (2009) argue:

> The workplace is no longer seen as the battleground between "capital" and "labour", it would be more accurate to say that the class war has become the "couch war" with both sides [employers and trade unions] trying to help employees onto the therapy couch.
>
> (Ecclestone and Hayes 2009: 105)

The suggestion of then government minister Norman Tebbit in 1981 to unemployed people that they get on their bikes and look for work was criticized at the time for individualizing a structural problem.[1] Today, it would be more likely to be seen as insensitive due to its assumption that such individuals could do so unaided by professional expertise. The equivalent injunction to unemployed people would be to 'get on the couch and be helped to look for work'.[2] Today, even those who 'survive' workplace redundancy and remain in their job are said to need counselling. According to Jonathan Naess, a consultant on workplace culture and mental health, 'careful framing and explanation [by employers] of why competent loyal employees are being forced out will be needed to preserve the "psychological contract" with those who remain' (Naess 2010: 6).

The rise of interest in the emotional health of the workforce is also beneficial to the employers. The mentally healthy 'stress-fit' worker is likely to be more productive, therefore 'the stress discourse conveniently conjoins individual and organizational health' (Newton 1995: 60). Newton backs up this argument by pointing out that company investment in 'stress management' consultants and initiatives increased during the 1980s, which was a time of labour surplus. Their input therefore could not have been about recruitment or retention of staff, but more to do with making the existing workforce more economically valuable by increasing their productivity. In fact the drive for employers to have stress management polices comes from all sides; from employees, trade unions, government and the human resource industry.

The establishment of a therapeutic discourse and health and safety legislation centred on worker vulnerability was not the only area in which the ranks of the 'vulnerable' were expanded, as can be illustrated by recent legal changes in what or who constitutes a 'vulnerable adult'.

The legal construction of the vulnerable adult[3]

Since the mid 1990s there has been a remarkable expansion in the number of people, both children and adults, who are now officially classed as vulnerable. According to the *Every Child Matters* policy document, there are approximately 11 million children living in England, between 3 and 4 million of whom are considered to be 'vulnerable', although the term is not defined (Department for Education and Skills (DFES) 2003). I wrote to the Department of Children, Schools and Families (DCSF) to ask how they defined 'vulnerable' and on what basis they could make such a claim, and was informed in reply that they had used 'a broad definition of vulnerability including vulnerability through living below the official poverty line' (personal communication, March 31, 2009). At a stroke a significant proportion of the nation's children were now officially vulnerable. However, it is in relation to the perception of adults that the construction of vulnerability and its expansion is most instructive, and can be illustrated by detailing the changes in legal definitions of what constitutes someone as a 'vulnerable adult'.

In 1995, the Law Commission proposed the following definition:

> a 'vulnerable person at risk' should mean any person of 16 or over who (1) is or may be in need of community care services by reason of mental or other disability, age or illness *and who* (2) is or may be unable to take care of himself or herself, or unable to protect himself or herself against *significant harm* or *serious exploitation*.
>
> (Law Commission 1995, my emphasis)

It is clear from this definition that vulnerability is not automatically assumed to flow from the specific categories mentioned. In addition, even being at risk of harm or exploitation is not sufficient for the label of vulnerable to be applied; the harm must be significant, the exploitation serious. No doubt such a high threshold was used to withhold services from people who needed it, but it also reflected a view that to be vulnerable was not considered the norm. This definition was adapted by the Lord Chancellor's Department in 1997, with 'vulnerable person' being replaced by 'vulnerable adult', and the word 'serious' was dropped to leave a similar threshold for harm and exploitation, both now being required to be 'significant'. This definition was adopted by most local authorities.

A mere three years later, the policy guidance document *No Secrets* (Department of Health (DH) 2000), while keeping the 1997 definition, elaborated on what constituted 'community care services' 'to include all care services in any setting or context' (para.2.4). However, the same year the Care Standards Act 2000 expanded the definition to a quite considerable extent. A 'vulnerable adult' was now

(a) an adult to whom accommodation and nursing or personal care are provided in a care home;
(b) an adult to whom personal care is provided in their own home under arrangements made by a domiciliary care agency; or
(c) an adult to whom prescribed services are provided by an independent hospital, independent clinic, independent medical agency or National Health Service body.
(Care Standards Act 2000, part VII, 6)

Gone is the need to belong to a specific category of service user, as is the need to be at risk of any form of harm or exploitation, never mind of a significant degree. Simply to use one such service now automatically classifies you as a vulnerable adult. While such a move was likely made with the best of intentions there is a sense that not only do they view such adults as lacking resilience, they also view those charged with caring for them as a source of risk.

The trend to further expand the category of 'vulnerable adult' continued, culminating in the Safeguarding Vulnerable Groups Act 2006, which views a person to be a vulnerable adult if they have attained the age of 18, and he or she

(a) is in residential accommodation
(b) is in sheltered housing
(c) receives domiciliary care
(d) receives any form of health care
(e) is detained in lawful custody
(f) is by virtue of an order of a court under supervision by a person exercising functions for the purposes of Part 1 of the Criminal Justice and Court Services Act 2000 (c.43)[4]
(g) receives a welfare service of a prescribed description[5]
(h) receives any service or participates in any activity provided specifically for persons who fall within subsection (9)[6]

   (i) payments are made to him (or to another on his behalf) in
        pursuance of arrangements under section 57 of the Health
        and Social Care Act 2001 (c.15),[7] or
   (j) requires assistance in the conduct of his affairs
                    (Safeguarding Vulnerable Groups Act 2006, s.59[1])

This is quite a remarkable expansion, especially when you consider
that health care means receiving 'treatment, therapy or palliative care
of *any* description' (s.59[5], my emphasis), while any provision of
assistance by virtue of age, health or any disability also renders the
recipient among the ranks of the vulnerable (s.59[5]).

As the vast majority of people with disabilities require some form
of assistance, to varying degrees and length of time, this legislation
effectively equates having a disability with being a 'vulnerable adult'.
With dyslexia now recognized as a form of disability, and with many
higher education students having assistance for just such a diagnosis,
the implication is that they are vulnerable adults also. However, in a
rare moment of insight into the absurdity of such a broad definition,
officials working for the Independent Safeguarding Authority (ISA)
specifically removed dyslexia-related services from the list of those to
be classified as 'vulnerable' (ISA 2008).

It is difficult to get precise figures for how many people are now
officially classed as vulnerable, due to the potential for overlap. Some
people will be in more than one category, for example receiving
community care and health services and/or being in lawful custody
and suffering mental health problems. Nevertheless, it is clear that at
some point in any given year, a majority of the UK adult population
would be labelled as 'vulnerable'. For example:

> In 2007–08, 1.77 million clients were in receipt of social care
> services, 1.53 million (87 per cent) of whom received community-
> based services.
> During a sample week in September 2008, 340,600 people
> received a total of 4.1 million contact hours of home care.
> 78% of people will see their GP at least once during the year. GPs
> also refer 14% of the population to hospital specialities.
> In 2008–09, over 1.2 million people accessed NHS mental health
> services.
> There were 85,086 detained prisoners as of 30 April 2010.
>   (McLaughlin and Appleton 2010: 14)

It is also worth noting the equating of being in 'lawful custody' with
being a vulnerable adult, which amounts to a sort of therapeutic

exposition of criminology. In addition, included under the category 'in lawful custody' is any

> detained person (within the meaning of Part 8 of the Immigration and Asylum Act 1999 (c.33)) who is detained in a removal centre or short term holding facility (within the meaning of that Part) or in pursuance of escort arrangements made under section 156 of that Act.
> (Safeguarding Vulnerable Groups Act 2006, s.59, s.7, d)

The terrain of the immigration debate has, in many respects, coalesced around vulnerability; the extent to which the asylum seeker has suffered physical or psychological harm having great bearing on whether their application to remain in the UK is successful or not. Whatever the outcome, the border authorities are presented as protectors of the vulnerable asylum seeker; either allowing them to stay in view of their trauma, or taking care of them during the removal process.

The changing debate around immigration is instructive in how Political issues (with a capital P) have been downgraded and replaced by a psychological approach, dominated by the micropolitical (politics with a small p). Those who wish to be granted rights of residence are obliged to adopt the role of traumatized victim. This presentation of the damaged self can be a pragmatically chosen identity by those seeking to remain in the UK, as they seek to overcome the legalistic hurdles that prevent the free movement of people across national borders. However, as macropolitical issues are downgraded, the subject of immigration is increasingly viewed as a non-political issue; the need for heavily restricted national borders becomes almost naturalized and the removal process becomes an instrumental one disconnected from issues of social justice.

This process of the depoliticization of immigration policy and practice, and its repositioning as a psychological issue, casts those subject to immigration control and detention as vulnerable, victims requiring protection and care while awaiting removal from the country. The asylum seeker is here constructed as automatically vulnerable with the border control agencies (which include psychologists and social workers) presented as their benefactors.

Protecting the vulnerable?

If a substantial proportion of the population are officially 'vulnerable', it follows that there is a need to protect them. In this respect the coalescence of all the major political parties around a politics based on fear and the inherent vulnerability of the population to physical or psychological trauma can lead to the expansion of state control over a significant section of the population. Presented as sensible measures to protect the vulnerable, the construction of vulnerability in its recent historical context is rarely considered. From the perspective of inherent vulnerability we are all considered at risk and therefore even the receipt of social care carries with it a risk of harm. Caring relationships are recast as ones of potential abuse and harm. They too become something to be survived. Indeed, it is this sense of heightened fear and vulnerability that has seen more and more relations of care become subject to state intrusion, for example via the expansion of criminal records checks for those working with, or coming into contact with, the newly expanded ranks of the 'vulnerable' (McLaughlin and Appleton 2010).

Prior to 2002, guidance for police checks was set out in Home Office Circular 47/93 (Home Office 1993) and covered people who applied for employment with local authorities or schools for work that would give them 'substantial unsupervised access, on a sustained or regular basis . . . to children under the age of sixteen'. With a significant section of the adult population now meeting the government's criteria to be classed as officially vulnerable, there has been a concomitant extension of vetting to those working with the 'vulnerable adult' population also. And, in line with developments for those working with children, not only those with 'substantial unsupervised access' to 'vulnerable adults' require vetting, but also any employee or volunteer whose duties may bring them into contact with such people.

For example, it is not even necessary to have any contact with a 'vulnerable person' to be required to undergo Criminal Records Bureau (CRB) clearance; merely having access to confidential information about children or vulnerable adults is sufficient for many organizations to require the vetting of their staff. In other cases, people are checked who have 'access to information about vulnerable adults', for example care records, or who do intellectual work on vulnerable adults, for example in social work academia. In a short space of time we have gone from viewing the need to vet staff as a rare event in very specific circumstances to one in which such vetting is ubiquitous.

Even drunk people can be classed as 'vulnerable adults'. A Christian organization that walks the streets helping drunken revellers at weekends requires its volunteers to be CRB checked, since they are helping the 'vulnerable'. In addition, homeless charities routinely

CRB check the volunteers who work in their shops, whose main activity is putting customers' items into carrier bags. Crisis, the homeless charity, CRB checks many of the volunteers who take food to people living on the streets around Christmas time. Age Concern Sussex advertised a 'befriender' scheme, which would include volunteers visiting an old person for 'general chatting or sharing hobbies such as crosswords and chess'. The Age Concern representative said that 'volunteers will need a CRB check' (McLaughlin and Appleton 2010: 7–8).

In addition to a CRB check, carers are also checked against the Protection of Vulnerable Adults (POVA) list. The POVA scheme was launched in July 2004, and laid down by section 80 of the Care Standards Act 2000. It is a system whereby 'known abusers' of vulnerable adults have their names put on a register. Section 80 of the Care Standards Act requires care agencies to refer a worker to the list if they have been suspended, sacked or moved to a non-care role because of evidence or suspicion that they have harmed a service user or placed them in danger.

Care providers and agencies in England and Wales have a statutory duty to consult the register whenever they employ someone whose work involves care duties for those considered vulnerable, and they cannot employ anyone whose name appears on the list. It is a criminal offence, punishable by up to five years in prison, for someone whose name appears on the list to seek employment in a care position. So, while the employer has the discretion to appoint someone with criminal convictions, they have no such discretion over anyone whose name is on the POVA list.

The rise of CRB checking of those working with 'vulnerable adults' can be illustrated by looking at the number of CRB applications received since 2002 where a check of the POVA list was also requested. The POVA list, formerly owned by the Department for Education and Skills, is now owned and maintained by the Independent Safeguarding Authority and is known as the ISA adults barred list.

Table 2 shows the number of CRB checks for those working or volunteering with vulnerable adults (i.e. where a POVA check was also requested as part of the CRB check). Even allowing for overlap, where the same person may have been POVA checked more than once, such figures indicate a massive expansion in the numbers of care employees and volunteers being vetted.

If current plans go ahead, a substantial number of adult carers would have to register on the vetting database. According to figures

Table 2 Criminal Record Bureau checks 2002–10

Year	CRB Checks	CRB checks for volunteers	CRB checks for non-volunteers
2002–03[a]	6	0	6
2003–04	29	1	28
2004–05	369,049	29,459	339,590
2005–06	516,062	45,729	470,333
2006–07	483,961	53,189	430,772
2007–08	487,441	54,789	432,652
2008–09	515,341	58,031	457,310
2009–10	568,877[b]	67,432	454,039
Total	*2,940,766*	*308,630*	*2,584,730*

Notes
a   Figures for 2002–09 from Manifesto Club Freedom of Information Act request to CRB, no. 14597.
b   Figures for 2009–10 from Manifesto Club Freedom of Information Act request to CRB, no. 14597. These figures were given for up to the end of February 2010, so have been scaled up proportionally to give cover until the end of March 2010.

from the CRB, released to the Manifesto Club, out of a total of 2 million volunteers who would have to register on the vetting database if it goes ahead as planned, around 500,000 of these would be volunteering with vulnerable adults.[8]

At the time of writing (April 2011), the new Conservative-Liberal coalition government is in the process of reviewing the vetting scheme with the aim of scaling back what has been seen to be an out of control process. The government's aim is to make such vetting necessary only when someone has 'close and frequent' contact with children or vulnerable adults, which they say will reduce the total number requiring to be vetted (workers and volunteers) from 11 million to 4 million. However, as well as lacking clarity, 'close and frequent' contact is not defined; such is the cultural strength of the risk/vulnerability nexus that almost immediately such measures were criticized for putting vulnerable people at risk from predators and paedophiles (Appleton 2011).

In addition, such discussions rarely consider my central point, that the current conceptualization of what constitutes a 'vulnerable adult' is a recent cultural construct, has broadened exponentially and is itself open to question.

Adults at risk?

The rationale for the above developments is to protect the 'vulnerable' from abuse. Nobody working in social work or social care would deny that some adults suffer serious and sustained abuse: such a position would be untenable. However, while provision must be made to protect people in such instances, it is not the case that there is an epidemic of abuse that requires a state monitoring system of all adult carers.

In 2007 the *UK Study of Abuse and Neglect* (O'Keeffe et al. 2007) found that 2.6 per cent of its sample of people aged 66 and over who lived in private households had 'experienced mistreatment' from a family member, close friend or care worker. This may include some horrific individual cases, but it does not suggest widespread mistreatment, especially when you consider that older people make up 72 per cent of social services' clients (National Health Service (NHS) 2010). In addition, there tends to be a conflation of categories in the way such reports are interpreted. A small number of very bad cases of abuse are listed alongside a more common form of mistreatment: 'neglect'. While the consequences of neglect can be serious, it is more often than not an act of omission rather than necessarily a calculated form of abuse.

Other forms of abuse, such as psychological, physical and sexual, were so uncommon that the report's authors combined them under the term 'interpersonal abuse'. The situation is further blurred by the wide range of behaviours included in some definitions. For instance, psychological abuse included such behaviours as shouting and taunting, which can certainly be unpleasant but are a long way from the serious end of the abuse spectrum.

Between July 2004 and November 2006, 3418 workers were referred for investigation for possible inclusion on the Protection of Vulnerable Adults list. Two-thirds of these were closed at the 'preprovisional' (first) stage of investigation and only 10.6 per cent were subsequently placed on the POVA list following further investigations (DH 2008). This would indicate two things. First, employers are referring staff too readily for POVA investigation, no doubt afraid not to comply with the procedures and face sanction themselves. Second, an average of 12 or 13 people a month being placed on the POVA list does not indicate widespread mistreatment of vulnerable people. And while it has to be borne in mind that some perpetrators may have escaped censure due to lack of evidence and/or credibility of a victim or witness, it is also the case that those who were deemed guilty were found so on the 'balance of probabilities', rather than the more stringent 'beyond reasonable doubt' legal threshold. This conclusion is also suggested if we examine the numbers of CRB checked adults who turned out to be on the adults barred list for the period

2009–10. Out of a total of 2.25 million CRB checks, only 89 were on the ISA adults barred list.[9]

The current expansion and incorporation of a discourse of inherent vulnerability, ubiquitous danger and risk-averse ethos into political and public life is a social construction, influenced to a significant degree by the trends discussed in earlier chapters. This manifests itself in bureaucratic, procedural attempts to reduce risk, such as the expansion of CRB checks for increasing numbers of the population. However, it has significant downsides. One is the erosion of important civil liberties protections, as endowed in the Rehabilitation of Offenders Act 1974. Another is the creation of a climate of mistrust that can further estrange us from one another, which can then feed back into our feelings of isolation and alienation. In this way, such procedural attempts to help the 'vulnerable', either by expanding the definition of the term or by emphasizing myriad potential threats to their welfare, actively constructs that which it then purports to protect.

Conclusion

If the demand for recognition increasingly articulated by contemporary social movements was predominantly one seeking affirmation of trauma and the vulnerable self, it is clear that such a mindset influences the discourse of both popular and mainstream political culture. In the realm of social policy, while there is a demand from below for initiatives that recognize the individual as one who is at risk and in need of protection, in many respects the imposition of a vulnerable identity is a top-down process, institutionalized within legislation and social policy.

Trade unions and numerous campaign groups articulate their needs as being due to the inherent weakness of those they claim to represent. Increasingly, social policy is based on a construction of the electorate as being comprised of vulnerable and/or abusive adults in need of state protection and control.

The dominance of a therapeutic and vulnerable identity, of a fragile self constantly at risk, not only undermines our relationships with each other, but also those with our employees and colleagues. Informal interactions, whether of a social or caring nature, are undermined when they are automatically viewed with suspicion until sanctioned by the state. Work conflict and disagreements are best resolved by responsible adults, not by therapists or by resorting to the language of the school playground.

Our relationship to government and the democratic process also changes. The concept of democracy rests on the assumption that we, as rational agents, elect and hold parliament to account. If, on the contrary, we are classed as irrational, as suffering from myriad mental disorders that limit our capacity and responsibility, as vulnerable adults unable to negotiate relationships, then the basis of democratic accountability is seriously compromised. Instead of 'we, the people' holding the state to account, the state takes on the role of doctor caring for a vulnerable, irrational and potentially dangerous electorate.

It is clear that the government, campaign groups and many mental health professionals (although there are also many who are deeply concerned by current developments) have a low opinion of people's ability to negotiate and transcend the problems of contemporary social and political life, and they have a vested interest in viewing us as sick and irrational. It should also be clear that allowing them to get away with this interpretation unchallenged poses a danger to our personal autonomy and political agency.

Notes

1 Tebbit actually said, in response to a question asking if the inner city riots of the time were not linked to rising unemployment, 'I grew up in the '30s with an unemployed father. He didn't riot. He got on his bike and looked for work, and he kept looking 'til he found it'. The common interpretation of this was that he was telling unemployed people to get on their bikes also.
2 It is worth noting that behind such public rhetoric it was actually the Conservative government of which Tebbit was a minister that introduced the offer of counselling for workers facing redundancy. Widely criticized at the time, it is something that is standard practice nowadays.
3 This section is developed from material discussed in my 2010 article 'Control and Social Work: A Reflection on Some Twenty-First Century Developments', *Practice*, 22(3): 143–154.
4 This refers to those subject to supervision by the probation service.
5 This includes services which provide support, assistance, advice or counselling to individuals with particular needs.
6 A person falls within this subsection if (a) he has particular needs because of his age; (b) he has any form of disability; (c) he has a physical or mental problem of such description as is prescribed; (d) she is an expectant or nursing mother in receipt of residential accommodation pursuant to arrangements made under section 21(1) (aa) of the National Assistance Act 1948 or care pursuant to paragraph 1 of Schedule 8 to the National Health Service Act 1977 (c. 49); (e) he is a person of a prescribed description not falling within paragraphs (a) to (d).
7 This refers to those in receipt of 'direct payments'.
8 CRB response to Manifesto Club FOI request, 29 April 2010.
9 Response to Manifesto Club FOI request to CRB, no. 16057.

Conclusion

The process of identity formation is a complex one. While experienced individually, identities are shaped by myriad interactions. It may be the case that we require our existence, our humanity, our identity, to be afforded recognition. However, if recognition is a vital human need, it is also a historically specific one, influenced by changes in the material world. Existing forms of individual and group identification have not come from nowhere. The rise of the therapeutic is not an inevitable process of modernization. The loss of authority and cultural meaning attached to the institutions and ideologies of modernity has certainly influenced the current situation, but this has been exacerbated by changing political attachments that at times betray anti-human sentiments and an implicit contempt for the public.

The discourse of psychology frames how political and interpersonal problems are discussed and conceptualized nowadays. In the workplace, traditional Marxist concerns over the tension between capital and labour, the process of alienation and exploitation due to the extraction of surplus value are rarely heard. Instead, they are replaced by the discourse of stress, bullying and counselling. As such, in the current period the demand for recognition not only takes on a specific psychological form but it is also framed within a therapeutic discourse of assumed vulnerability. Given the ubiquitous toxic agents that are said to be hazardous to our health, both physical and mental, it is conceivably no mean feat just to survive today. It is perhaps no surprise, then, that in addition to the imposition of a vulnerable identity from professionals and policymakers, more and more of us are also willing to define ourselves as vulnerable.

As we have seen, the field of political struggle has changed significantly in recent times. Class politics and struggle no longer dominate the political sphere. The mass political movements of the twentieth century have been replaced by new social movements that are more concerned with cultural and lifestyle issues than with economic redistribution. There has been an evacuation of the masses from political life, the vacuum filled by a new breed of middle and upper class dominated organizations. A therapeutic mode of understanding permeates all echelons of society. The politics of recognition, in interaction with wider political and social change, has become heavily focused on the fragility of the self, inherent vulnerability and susceptibility to psychological and physical harm.

As a defining political demand of the contemporary period, claims for recognition are no longer solely concerned with social justice issues, for example around misrecognition on account of gender, sexuality, ethnicity or disability. Instead, they often take the form of recognition of individual distress. Despite attempts by many to highlight the social and political aspects around issues of sexual and physical violence, where those of a more radical persuasion call into question the legitimacy of existing social relations, such endeavours can be reduced to the purely personal or interpersonal realm. This not only absolves the system from any culpability but also allows the state to be recast as benign carer to the traumatized and vulnerable victim.

The concept of trauma no longer refers to extreme experiences but has become normalized. The public expression of trauma has also gone mainstream and with it the expansion of the concept of 'survivor', as social movements increasingly focus on the psychological hurt being suffered by both the individual and the group. From the horrific experiences of the Holocaust, the term 'survivor' is now used liberally and can refer to a vast array of unpleasant experiences that bear little relation to what the Nazi death camp victims and survivors suffered.

There has been the emergence of a political outlook that increasingly is inward directed towards the self. The self can be the main, if not the sole reference point. When Holocaust and abuse survivor narratives accede to professional expertise, it is often to those who seek not to dispute it but to analyse, diagnose and formulate a treatment plan – the deference is to the psy-disciplines rather than sociologists or historians. For those who identify as 'psychiatric survivors', many of whom are extremely hostile to such professionals and who dispute that such practitioners hold any scientific or medical expertise whatsoever, the psy-disciplines are part of the problem not part of the solution. Nevertheless, while narratives of 'illness' as explanation for mental distress and/or psychotic phenomena are disputed, the framework of past abuse and trauma still locates them within a predominantly therapeutic rather than a historical material concept of alienation and distress.

The Movement for Happiness: a very modern social movement[1]

With so much focus on unhappiness, it is perhaps no surprise to find government and policymakers looking at ways to improve our psychological health, and maybe it was only a matter of time before someone came up with the idea of starting a movement devoted to increasing our levels of happiness.

As people attempt to make sense of their experiences, to give them meaning, they do so via the available frameworks and paradigms of the age, which are historically specific and imbued with political power and conflict. Today, the dominant paradigms are infused with identity politics and recognition of cultural difference, and often framed around psychiatric and psychological categories. As we have seen, many social movement activists and theorists have played a part in cultivating this sense of vulnerability, of the need for past trauma to be validated as authentic and afforded public recognition.

Likewise, trade unions have also resorted to the use of such a discourse as they seek to reposition themselves in relation to their members and employers at a time when their collective powers have significantly diminished. The political establishment also promotes the language of therapy in relation to growing numbers of seemingly intractable social and political problems. The debate over the 2010 proposed cuts to welfare benefits reduces the issue of unemployment to an individual level; it is caused either by the illness and/or moral fecklessness of those out of work. Prior to losing the 2010 general election, the New Labour government proposed cognitive behaviour therapy (CBT) as a strategy to combat long term unemployment; counselling sessions at the job centre are seen as a way of helping unemployed people back into the workforce (Stratton 2009). CBT is also championed as a way to combat such things as alcohol and drug misuse, depression and anxiety. When you consider how embedded alcohol is within British culture and the complex reasons for over-indulgence by some, the idea that this can be changed by six or seven sessions with a counsellor shows both naivety and a lack of political imagination by the proponents of such initiatives.

If anything, such trends are likely to continue for some time. Indeed, a highly symbolic new movement, in that it reflects the pre-vailing mood of the times, is the Movement for Happiness set up by

Lord Richard Layard, labelled the 'happiness tsar' when appointed by the then New Labour government to look at ways of improving the mental well-being of the populace, Geoff Mulgan, founder of the think-tank *Demos* and former Head of Policy in the Prime Minister's office during the New Labour years, and the political historian Anthony Seldon. In 2006 Layard proposed the training of an additional 10,000 CBT therapists, who were to be based in 250 centres across the UK. It remains to be seen whether the new Conservative-Liberal coalition government go ahead with this due to the scale of cuts to state-funded services (although Layard argues his proposal would be cost-effective as it would get sick people back to work), but current Prime Minister David Cameron is also concerned about the mental health of the nation, commenting that 'there's more to life than money and it's time we focused not just on GDP [Gross Domestic Product] but on GWB – general well-being' (quoted in Stratton 2010).[2]

Layard, in a lecture delivered to the London School of Economics in 2003, uses the following quote by Marx to back up a point he is making that our wants are largely derived from society: 'A house may be large or small; as long as the surrounding houses are equally small, it satisfies all social demands for a dwelling. But if a palace rises beside the little house, the little house shrinks into a hut' (quoted in Layard 2003: 13). However, Layard's analysis is certainly not a Marxist materialist one, and his conclusions are similar to those of other movement theorists today. His aim is not to have palaces for all but to make people happy in their huts, a sentiment that would no doubt find favour with many environmental activists concerned with unfettered materialism.

Layard's Movement for Happiness aims to become

> a mass movement, eventually worldwide in scope . . . Its members will commit themselves to trying to produce more happiness in the world and less misery. This will apply to their private lives, in how they are at work, and in what they do in the community – including the policies they ask policy-makers to adopt.
>
> (Layard et al. 2010)

These potential worldwide policies are very much concerned with equality, but the type of inequality prioritized for rectification is not of the economic variety.[3] The movement's founders inform us that

We can surely create a society in which people feel better inside themselves – where they are happier. Such a society has to start with individuals and their goals. But it also has to provide the external context in which all people can flourish –*social justice means a world without excessive inequalities in happiness*.
(Layard et al. 2010, my emphasis)

For Layard, the emphasis is on the psychological and emotional over the material, with lifestyle and cultural concerns over economic ones, with recognition rather than redistribution. With its not so subtle belief that the population require the beneficence of enlightened betters, and its assumption that we are all vulnerable to trauma, it could be argued that this new social movement represents the natural synthesis of the psychologization of social and political life, the downgrading of materialism and contempt for the public that is evident within much contemporary social movement theory and practice. The happiness movement, like many of the new social movements, is middle and upper class dominated, and while its members are clearly not on the margins of the political establishment, such a disjuncture is also increasingly blurred within many contemporary movements. In addition, its three founding fathers may be numerically insignificant but they inhabit a culture all too ready to give credence to their views: after all, as was discussed in Chapter 3, the original second-generation Holocaust survivors' meeting is reported to have had only five attendees.

The Movement for Happiness's manifesto cites figures that show that since the 1960s, the number of people answering 'yes' when asked the question 'Do you think most other people can be trusted?' has declined from 60 to 30 per cent. This is a problem because 'For a happier society we have to turn this tide of narrow individualism – as we all know, the greatest enemy of happiness is pre-occupation with the self' (Layard et al. 2010).

Here, Layard et al. (2010) have a point. There has been a loss of faith and trust within contemporary society. This is not confined to a decline in religious belief in an increasingly secular society; its effects go much wider than that, permeating many other social institutions as well as the intellectual and political traditions across the old divide between Left and Right. The authority of politicians and political parties has been eroded in recent years. The percentage of eligible voters actually casting a vote remains low. The view of much of the electorate is that political figures are out of touch with the people, are corrupt and cannot be trusted. The parliamentary expenses scandal of

2009, when many Members of Parliament were found to be claiming for dubious 'second homes', garden maintenance and even pornographic films seemed to confirm that they were in politics not because of their beliefs or on behalf of their constituents but solely for their own gain, in terms of the financial, career and status benefits they could accrue. Such cynicism starts young, one report finding that by the time they reach 18 years of age, one-third of those polled said they do not trust politicians 'at all' (cited in *Guardian* 23 November 2010).

Other institutions such as the church have also suffered, not only from declining congregations but also from child abuse scandals that have undermined its authority at best, and implicated it in the covering up of such abuse at worst. So, the erosion of trust within society is a problem. Fears over the abuse of both children and adults has led to a situation where all those working or volunteering to help in the community are treated with suspicion and subject to a criminal records check before being allowed to engage in civic duty.

The irony of their concern about the lack of trust is that both Layard and Mulgan were senior advisers to New Labour during its time in government, and, as we discussed in Chapter 6, it was that period that witnessed an exponential expansion of the concept of vulnerability and rise in criminal records checks for numerous social interactions. Both trends stem from the government's lack of trust in the population, which is viewed as weak, at risk and/or potential predators. Indeed, civil society, that sphere of voluntary social engagement lying between the public and private spheres, has effectively been colonized by the state and its intermediaries to such an extent that rather than being autonomous, organic entities responding to local need, such groups are often co-opted into implementing government policy by proxy (Hodgson 2004).

The rise of the new social movements, in many respects, was also influenced by a loss of faith, in modernity, progress and the historical subject, and the way in which the working class went from being viewed as the agents of the revolutionary change of society, to being seen as people who required educating by their middle class 'betters' in order to eradicate their prejudices. Such disdain for the masses is seldom overtly expressed but is evident in, for example, the way many environmentalists rail against cheap air flights, or if put more bluntly, at the way flight prices are now so low that the working classes can also afford to holiday abroad. Similarly, latter day evangelicals, such as the celebrity chef Jamie Oliver, may set out with the best of intentions, but when the masses fail to heed their sage advice on how to improve their unhealthy dietary habits, a contemptuous side becomes evident as, in Oliver's case, the unconvinced are berated as 'arseholes' and 'tossers' (Cassidy 2006). More subtle forms of the expression of disdain are also evident in the assumption that people are inherently vulnerable and potentially dangerous.

In this sense, perhaps Layard's movement is not as absurd as it appears at first glance. On the contrary, it may represent the logical outcome of the trajectory of late twentieth century political thought, aided not only by capitalist enterprise and neo-liberal ideology but also, to a considerable extent, by those on the political left, whose disillusionment with the history-making potential of the masses led to an inward turn to the self, to the search for 'socialism in one person' rather than in society. Rather than being an aberration, a happiness movement reflects perfectly the zeitgeist of our times.

The degraded subject of new social movements

The demise of the labour movement, and with it the strength of the trade unions, may have allowed for the easier exploitation of the workforce by employers, and allowed neo-liberal economic policies to be implemented by the political establishment, but there was a price to be paid for this victory. For the political elite, the trade union movement gave them a link to the masses, an opportunity to connect at some level with their concerns and desires. Given the decline of the old movements and their replacement by middle class dominated ones this link no longer exists to the same degree as in the past. There is a vacuum between those who govern and those that are governed.

With the loss of a political, historical subject, of agents of social change, the new social movements are, as Melucci (1988) and Offe (1987) acknowledge, essentially conservative in nature. For Melucci (1988: 254), 'the central problem of complex systems is the main-tenance of equilibrium'. With their defence of cultural traditions and identities there is an antagonism towards the concept of linear progress. As Heartfield (2002) notes, at heart many of the new social movements have been revealed as not being *social* movements at all. Rather, 'the underlying dynamic was always conservative and elite politics, though that could only gain full expression with the defeat of the organised labour movement in the eighties' (Heartfield 2002: 153).

The conservatism inherent in the new social movements, their desire for preservation, applies not only society but also the individual psyche. With social change increasingly off the agenda, the focus is on individual growth, a 'revolution from within', on repairing the damage caused by alienation, not by changing the causes of alienation but by addressing its symptoms.

The rise in both individuals and groups that identify as survivors today is the result of many intertwined factors such as the psychologization of politics and the social world, a societal outlook that is increasingly past rather than future oriented, public estrangement from the political process and a public discourse of vulnerability and risk. However, these self-identified survivors are only the more public voice of the survivor ethos. The trends identified in this book affect us all. By lowering our expectations of ourselves and each other, the prevailing mood is one in which we are all survivors, not necessarily of genuinely traumatic events but of everyday life itself. Personal, social and political problems are seen as beyond our control, the best we can hope for is to cope with rather than transcend them. Such an outlook needs to be challenged. To survive should not be seen as our goal; the point of life is not to survive but to live, to become. There is, therefore, an urgent need to reclaim the historical subject, to view ourselves as the makers not the objects of history.

Notes

1 There were those within the psychology community promoting this idea since at least the 1950s, but it is in the twenty-first century that they have moved from within the discipline to wider society and also gained wider political appeal.

2 Political and intellectual concern with happiness is not new. For example, Aristotle, John Stuart Mill, Thomas Jefferson, Adam Smith and even Joseph Stalin gave it some thought. However, here I am locating Layard and colleagues' movement as a historically specific and debased manifestation of both the idea and the pursuit of happiness.

3 Economic issues do remain central to the Movement for Happiness in some respects, it being reported that they are looking to appoint a director on a salary of £80,000 per annum (Low 2010).

References

Abercrombie, N., Hill, S. and Turner, B.S. (2006) *The Penguin Dictionary of Sociology*, London: Penguin.

Alcoff, L. and Gray, L. (1993) 'Survivor Discourse: Transgression or Recuperation?', *Signs: Journal of Women and Society*, 18: 260–290.

Allott, P. (2000) *The Concept of Recovery in Mental Health*, Birmingham: Change.

Althusser, L. (1971) 'Ideology and Ideological State Apparatuses (Notes Towards an Investigation)', in Althusser, L., *Lenin and Philosophy and Other Essays*, New York: Monthly Review Press.

American Psychiatric Association (APA) (1952) *Diagnostic and Statistical Manual of Mental Disorders* (DSM-I), Washington, DC: APA.

American Psychiatric Association (APA) (1968) *Diagnostic and Statistical Manual of Mental Disorders* (DSM-II), Washington, DC: APA.

American Psychiatric Association (APA) (1980) *Diagnostic and Statistical Manual of Mental Disorders* (DSM-III), Washington, DC: APA.

American Psychiatric Association (APA) (1987) *Diagnostic and Statistical Manual of Mental Disorders* (DSM-III-R), Washington, DC: APA.

American Psychiatric Association (APA) (1994) *Diagnostic and Statistical Manual of Mental Disorders* (DSM-IV), Washington, DC: APA.

American Psychiatric Association (APA) (2000) *Diagnostic and Statistical Manual of Mental Disorders* (DSM-IV-TR), Washington, DC: APA.

Appiah, K.A. (1994) 'Identity, Authenticity, Survival: Multicultural Societies and Social Reproduction', in Gutmann, A. (ed.) *Multiculturalism: Examining the Politics of Recognition*, Oxford: Oxford University Press.

Appleton, J. (2011) 'Who are the 4 Million Who Will Have to be Vetted?', Manifesto Club. Available at www.manifestoclub.com/node/717 (accessed 12 April 2011).

Baghramian, A. and Kershaw, S. (1989) 'We are All Survivors like our Children', *Social Work Today*, 20(48): 20–21.

Barham, P. and Hayward, R. (1995) *Relocating Madness: From the Mental Patient to the Person*, London: Free Association Books.

Barnes, M. and Bowl, R. (2001) *Taking Over the Asylum: Empowerment and Mental Health*, Basingstoke: Palgrave.

Barnes, M. and Shardlow, P. (1997) 'From Passive Recipient to Active Citizen: Participation in Mental Health User Groups', *Journal of Mental Health*, 6: 289–300.

Barnett, S. (2008) 'Bonkersfest', *New Statesman*, 8 July. Available at www. newstatesman.com/print/200807080005 (accessed 14 September 2010).

Bean, K. (2007) *The New Politics of Sinn Fein*, Liverpool: Liverpool University Press.

Beck, U. (1992) *Risk Society: Towards a New Modernity*, London: Sage.

Benhabib, S. (1992) *Situating the Self: Gender, Community and Postmodernism in Contemporary Ethics*, London: Routledge.

Benhabib, S. (1995) 'Feminism and Postmodernism: An Uneasy Alliance', in Benhabib, S., Butler, J., Cornell, D., Fraser, N. and Nicholson, L. (eds) *Feminist Contentions: A Philosophical Exchange*, London: Routledge.

Benhabib, S., Butler, J., Cornell, D., Fraser, N. and Nicholson, L. (eds) (1995) *Feminist Contentions: A Philosophical Exchange*, London: Routledge.

Beresford, P. and Wallcraft, J. (1997) 'Psychiatric System Survivors and Emancipatory Research: Issues, Overlaps and Differences', in Barnes, C. and Mercer, G. (eds) *Doing Disability Research*, Leeds: Disability Press.

Beresford, P., Glifford, G. and Harrison, C. (2000) 'What has Disability Got to Do with Psychiatric Survivors', in Read, J. and Reynolds, J. (eds) *Speaking our Minds: An Anthology*, Basingstoke: Palgrave.

Blashfield, R. and Fuller, K (1996) 'Predicting the DSM-V', *Journal of Nervous and Mental Disease*, 184: 4–7.

Bourdieu, P. (1977) *Outline of a Theory of Practice*, Cambridge: Cambridge University Press.

Bourdieu, P. (1993) *Sociology in Question*, London: Sage.

Bourdieu, P. and Wacquant, L. (1992) *An Investigation to Reflexive Sociology*, trans. Wacquant, L., Cambridge: Polity.

Brandon, D., Wells, K., Francis, C. and Ramsay, E. (1980) *The Survivors: A Study of Homeless Young Newcomers to London and the Responses to Them*, Henley-on-Thames: Routledge & Kegan Paul.

Bree, M.H. (1970) 'Staying the Course', *British Journal of Psychiatric Social Work*, 10(4): 170–177.

Breggin, P. (1991) *Toxic Psychiatry*, New York: St Martin's Press.

Browne, D. (1990) *Black People, Mental Health and the Courts*, London: Nacro.

Burke, E. (1993 [1790]) *Reflections on the Revolution in France*, Oxford: Oxford University Press.

Burman, E. (1996–97) 'False Memories, True Hopes and the Angelic: Revenge of the Postmodern in Therapy', *New Formations*, 30: 122–134.

Burstow, B. (2003) 'Toward a Radical Understanding of Trauma and Trauma Work', *Violence Against Women*, 9(11): 1293–1317.

Butler, J. (1990) *Gender Trouble: Feminism and the Subversion of Identity*, London: Routledge.

Butler, J. (2004) *Undoing Gender*, London: Routledge.

Butler, J. (2008) 'Merely Cultural', in Fraser, N., *Adding Insult to Injury: Nancy Fraser Debates her Critics* (edited by K. Olsen), London: Verso.

Campbell, P. (1992) 'A Survivor's View of Community Psychiatry', *Journal of Mental Health*, 1(2): 117–122.

Campbell, P. (1996) 'The History of the User Movement in the United Kingdom', in Heller, T., Reynolds, J., Gomm, R., Muston, R. and Pattison, S. (eds) *Mental Health Matters: A Reader*, London: Macmillan.

Campbell, P. (2010) 'Survivors Speak Out'. Available at http://studymore.org.uk/mpu.htm#SurvivorsSpeakOut (accessed 2 August 2010).

Canning, C. (2006) 'Psychiatric Survivor Testimonials and Embodiment: Emotional Challenges to Medical Knowledge', *Radical Psychology*, 1. Available at http://radicalpsychology.org/vol5/Canning.html (accessed 11 February 2010).

Capstone Report (2001) *Psychiatric Survivor Oral Histories: Implications for Contemporary Mental Health Policy*, Center for Public Policy and Administration, University of Massachusetts, Amherst, MA. Available at www.freedom-center.org/pdf/oryxpsychoralhistory.pdf (accessed 23 July 2011).

Carey, J. (1992) *The Intellectuals and the Masses: Pride and Prejudice Among the Literary Intelligentsia, 1880–1939*, London: Faber & Faber.

Cassidy, S. (2006) 'Jamie Oliver Rages Against "Crime" of Junk-Food Diets', *The Independent*, 8 September. Available at www.independent.co.uk/lifestyle/health-and-families/health-news/jamie-oliver-rages-against-crime-of-junkfood-diets-415089.html (accessed 22 November 2010).

Cesarani, D. (2001) 'Memory, Representation and Education', in Roth, J.K. and Maxwell, E. (eds) *Remembering for the Future: The Holocaust in an Age of Genocide*, New York: Palgrave.

Chamberlin, J. (1978) *On our Own: Patient Controlled Alternatives to the Mental Health System*, New York: McGraw-Hill.

Chamberlin, J. (1990) 'The Ex-Patient's Movement: Where We've Been and Where We're Going', *Journal of Mind and Behaviour*, 11: 323–336.

Chantler, K., Gangoli, G. and Hester, M. (2009) 'Forced Marriage in the UK: Religious, Cultural, Economic or State Violence', *Critical Social Policy*, 29(4): 587–612.

Chesler, P. (1972) *Women and Madness*, New York: Doubleday.

Chodoff, P. (1997) 'The Holocaust and its Effects on Survivors: An Overview', *Political Psychology*, 18(1): 147–157.

Cloud, D.L. (1998) *Control and Consolation in American Culture and Politics: Rhetoric of Therapy*, London: Sage.

Cohen, B.B. (2007) *Case Closed: Holocaust Survivors in Postwar America*, New Brunswick, NJ: Rutgers University Press.

Coleman, R. (1996) 'The Construction of Psychiatric Authority', *Asylum: The Magazine for Democratic Psychiatry*, 10(1): 11–15.

Collins, S., Gutridge, P., James, A., Lyn, E. and Williams, C. (2000) 'Racism and Anti-Racism in Placement Reports', *Social Work Education*, 19(1): 29–43.

Cook, K. and Kelly, L. (1997) 'The Abduction of Credibility: A Reply to John Paley', *British Journal of Social Work*, 27: 71–84.

Cooper, C. and Cartwright, S. (1994) 'Stress-Management Interventions in the Workplace: Stress Counselling and Stress Audits', *British Journal of Guidance and Counselling*, 22: 65–73.

Cotgrove, S. and Duff, A. (2003) 'Middle-Class Radicalism and Environmentalism', in Goodwin, J. and Jasper, J.M. (eds) *The Social Movements Reader: Cases and Concepts*, Oxford: Blackwell.

Crossley, M.L. and Crossley, N. (2001) '"Patient" Voices, Social Movements and the Habitus: How Psychiatric Survivors "Speak Out"', *Social Science and Medicine*, 52: 1477–1489.

Crossley, N. (1998) 'Transforming the Mental Health Field: The Early History of the National Association for Mental Health', *Sociology of Health and Illness*, 20: 458–488.

Crossley, N. (1999) 'Fish, Field, Habitus and Madness: The First Wave Mental Health Users Movement in Great Britain', *British Journal of Sociology*, 50(4): 647–670.

Crossley, N. (2002a) *Making Sense of Social Movements*, Maidenhead: Open University Press.

Crossley, N. (2002b) 'Repertoires of Contention and Tactical Diversity in the UK Psychiatric Survivors Movement: The Question of Appropriation', *Social Movement Studies*, 1(1): 47–71.

Crossley, N. (2006) *Contesting Psychiatry: Social Movements in Mental Health*, London: Routledge.

Dain, N. (1994) 'Psychiatry and Anti-Psychiatry in the United States', in Micale, M.S. and Porter, R. (eds) *Discovering the History of Psychiatry*, Oxford: Oxford University Press.

Danieli, Y. (ed.) (1998) *Intergenerational Handbook of Multigenerational Legacies of Trauma*, New York: Plenum.

Deegan, P.E. (1992) 'The Independent Living Movement and People with Psychiatric Disabilities: Taking Back Control Over our Lives', *Psychosocial Rehabilitation Journal*, 15(3): 3–19.

DeGloma, T.E. (undated) '"Safe Space" and Contested Memories: Survivor Movements and the Foundation of Alternative Mnemonic Traditions'. Available at www.newschool.edu/nssr/historymatters/papers/ThomasDeGloma.pdf (accessed 23 July 2011).

Department for Education and Skills (DfES) (2003) *Every Child Matters*, London: DfES. Available at www.education.gov.uk/consultations/downloadableDocs/EveryChildMatters.pdf (accessed 23 July 2011).

Department of Health (DH) (2000) *No Secrets: Guidance on Developing and Implementing Multi-Agency Policies and Procedures to Protect Vulnerable Adults from Abuse*, London: Department of Health.

140   *References*

Department of Health (DH) (2008) *The Protection of Vulnerable Adults List: An Investigation of Referral Patterns and Approaches to Decision Making.* Available at www.dh.gov.uk/prod_consum_dh/groups/dh_digitalassets/@dh/@en/documents/digitalasset/dh_086637.pdf (accessed 15 April 2010).

Des Pres, T. (1980) *The Survivor: An Anatomy of Life in the Death Camps*, Oxford: Oxford University Press.

Dineen, T. (1999) *Manufacturing Victims*, London: Constable.

Dominelli, L. (2002) *Anti-Oppressive Social Work Theory and Practice*, Basingstoke: Palgrave.

Durocher, N. (1999) 'Insights from Cult Survivors Regarding Group Support', *British Journal of Social Work*, 29: 581–599.

Eaglestone, R. (2004) *The Holocaust and the Postmodern*, Oxford: Oxford University Press.

Eatock, J. (2000) 'Counselling in Primary Care: Past, Present and Future', *British Journal of Guidance and Counselling*, 28: 161–173.

Ecclestone, K. and Hayes, D. (2009) *The Dangerous Rise of Therapeutic Education*, Abingdon: Routledge.

Edwards, G. (2004) 'Habermas and Social Movements: What's "New"?', *Sociological Review*, 52: 113–130.

Einwohner, R.L. (2007) 'Availability, Proximity, and Identity in the Warsaw Ghetto Uprising: Adding a Sociological Lens to Studies of Jewish Resistance', in Gregson, J.M. and Wolf, D.L. (eds) *Sociology Confronts the Holocaust: Memories and Identities in Jewish Diasporas*, Durham, NC: Duke University Press.

Epstein, H. (1988) *Children of the Holocaust: Conversations with Sons and Daughters of Survivors*, London: Penguin.

Evans, P. (1993) *Verbal Abuse Survivors Speak Out: On Relationship and Recovery*, Holbrook, MA: Bob Adams.

Evans, P. (undated) 'Frequently Asked Questions about Verbal Abuse'. Available at http://silverreflection.tripod.com/speakoutagainstverbalabuse copy/id8.html (accessed 7 April 2008).

Everett, B. (1994) 'Something is Happening: The Contemporary Consumer and Psychiatric Survivor Movement in Historical Context', *Journal of Mind and Behaviour*, 15: 55–57.

Eyerman, R. (2001) *Cultural Trauma: Slavery and the Formation of African American Identity*, New York: Cambridge University Press.

Faulkner, A. (2004) *The Ethics of Ethical Conduct of Research Carried Out by Mental Health Service Users and Survivors*, Bristol: Policy Press.

Feminists for Life of America (FFL) (2008) 'Abortion: The Second Rape'. Available at www.feministsforlife.org/FFL_topics/victory/2ndrape.htm (accessed 20 September 2010).

Fermaglich, K. (2003) 'The Comfortable Concentration Camp: The Significance of Nazi Imagery in Betty Friedan's The Feminine Mystique', *American Jewish History*, 91(2): 205–232.

Fernando, S. (2010) *Mental Health, Race and Culture*, Basingstoke: Palgrave.

Field, T. (1996) *Bullying in Sight: How to Predict, Resist, Challenge and Combat Workplace Bullying*, Didcot: Success Unlimited.

Finkelstein, N. (2000) *The Holocaust Industry: Reflections on the Exploitation of Jewish Suffering*, London: Verso.

Fitzgerald, M. (2009) 'Climate Change is a Feminist Issue', *Guardian*, Comment is Free. Available at www.guardian.co.uk/commentisfree/cif-green/2009/oct/27/climate-change-contraception-women-feminism (accessed 4 June 2010).

Fitzpatrick, M. (2001) *The Tyranny of Health: Doctors and the Regulation of Lifestyle*, London: Routledge.

Foucault, M. (1967) *Madness and Civilization: A History of Insanity in the Age of Reason*, London: Tavistock.

Foucault, M. (1972) *The Archaeology of Knowledge*, New York: Pantheon.

Foucault, M. (1979) *The History of Sexuality* (vol. 1), New York: Pantheon.

Foucault, M. (1980) *Power/Knowledge: Selected Interviews and Other Writings, 1972–1977*, New York: Pantheon.

Fraser, N. (1995) 'From Redistribution to Recognition: Dilemmas of Justice in a "Post-Socialist" Age', *New Left Review*, 212: 68–93.

Fraser, N. (2008) 'Why Overcoming Prejudice is Not Enough', in Fraser, N., *Adding Insult to Injury: Nancy Fraser Debates her Critics* (edited by K. Olsen), London: Verso.

Fraser, N. and Honneth, A. (2003) *Redistribution or Recognition: A Political-Philosophical Exchange*, London: Verso.

Friedan, B. (1986 [1963]) *The Feminine Mystique*, Harmondsworth: Penguin.

Fukuyama, F. (1992) *The End of History and the Last Man*, London: Penguin.

Furedi, F. (1997) *Culture of Fear: Risk-Taking and the Morality of Low Expectation*, London: Cassell.

Furedi, F. (2004) *Therapy Culture: Cultivating Vulnerability in an Uncertain Age*, London: Routledge.

General Whitley Council (GWC) (2000) 'Equal Opportunities Agreement', Advance Letter (GC) 1/2000.

Gerson, J.M. (2007) 'In Cuba I Was a German Shepherd: Questions of Comparison and Generalizability in Holocaust Memoirs', in Gerson, J.M. and Wolf, D.L. (eds) *Sociology Confronts the Holocaust: Memories and Identities in Jewish Diasporas*, Durham, NC: Duke University Press.

Gerson, J.M. and Wolf, D.L. (2007) 'Why Sociology? Why the Holocaust? Why Now?', in Gerson, J.M. and Wolf, D.L. (eds) *Sociology Confronts the Holocaust: Memories and Identities in Jewish Diasporas*, Durham, NC: Duke University Press.

Giddens, A. (1990) *The Consequences of Modernity*, Cambridge: Polity.

Giddens, A. (1997) *Sociology*, Cambridge: Polity.

Gilfus, M.E. (1999) 'The Price of the Ticket: A Survivor-Centred Appraisal of Trauma Theory', *Violence Against Women*, 5(11): 1238–1257.

Glendenning, C. (1994) *My Name is Chellis and I'm in Recovery from Western Civilization*, Boston, MA: Shambhala.

Goffman, E. (1961) *Asylums: Essays on the Social Situation of Mental Patients and Other Inmates*, Harmondsworth: Penguin.

Goldacre, B. (2009) *Bad Science*, London: HarperCollins.

Goldstrom, I.D., Campbell, J., Rogers, J.A., Lambert, D.B., Blacklow, B., Henderson, M.J. and Manderschied, R.W. (2006) 'National Estimates for Mental Health Mutual Support Groups, Self-Help Organizations and Consumer-Operated Services', *Administration and Policy in Mental Health and Mental Health Services Research*, 33: 92–102.

Goodwin, J. and Jasper, J.M. (2004) 'Caught in a Winding Snarling Vine: The Structural Bias of Political Process Theory', in Goodwin, J. and Jasper, J.M. (eds) *Rethinking Social Movements: Structure, Meaning and Emotion*, Oxford: Rowman & Littlefield.

Gottleib, R.S. (1994) 'Ethics and Trauma: Levinas, Feminism and Deep Ecology', *Cross Currents*, 44(2): 222–241. Available at www.crosscurrents.org/feministecology.htm (accessed 23 July 2011).

Gould, D.B. (2004) 'Passionate Political Processes: Bringing Emotions Back into the Study of Social Movements', in Goodwin, J. and Jasper, J.M. (eds) *Rethinking Social Movements: Structure, Meaning and Emotion*, Oxford: Rowman & Littlefield.

Green, B. (2004) 'Post-Traumatic Stress Disorder in UK Police Officers', *Current Medical Research and Opinion*, 20(1): 1–5. Available at www.greenmedicolegal.com/PTSDPOLICE.pdf (accessed 15 October 2010).

Haaken, J. (1998) *Pillar of Salt: Gender, Memory and the Perils of Looking Back*, New Brunswick, NJ: Rutgers University Press.

Habermas, J. (1981) 'New Social Movements', *Telos*, 49: 33–37.

Habermas, J. (1987) *Theory of Communicative Action: System and Lifeworld*, Cambridge: Polity.

Heartfield, J. (2002) *The 'Death of the Subject' Explained*, Sheffield: Sheffield Hallam University Press.

Heartfield, J. (2009) 'Radicalism Against the Masses', in Pugh, J. (ed.) *What is Radical Politics Today?* Basingstoke: Palgrave.

Hehir, B. (2004) 'The Pregnancy Police', *spiked*. Available at www.spiked-online.com, 3 November 2004 (accessed 4 April 2006).

Herman, J.L. (1992) *Trauma and Recovery*, New York: Basic Books.

Hirsch, M. (1997) *Family Frames: Photographs, Narrative and Postmemory*, London: Harvard University Press.

Hodgson, L. (2004) 'Manufactured Civil Society: Counting the Cost', *Critical Social Policy*, 24(2): 139–164.

Home Office (1993) *Protection of Children: Disclosure of Criminal Background of Those with Access to Children*, Home Office Circular no. 47/1993, London: HMSO.

Honneth, A. (2003) 'Redistribution as Recognition: A Response to Nancy Fraser', in Fraser, N. and Honneth, A., *Redistribution or Recognition: A Political-Philosophical Exchange*, London: Verso.

House of Lords (1998) *Judgments – White and Others v. Chief Constable of*

South Yorkshire and Others. Available at www.publications.parliament.uk/pa/ld199899/ldjudgmt/jd981203/white01.htm (accessed 25 October 2010).

Hume, M. (2010) 'Shock News: It's Not 1979 – or 1990', *spiked*. Available at www.spiked-online.com/index.php/site/article/9555/ (accessed 20 September 2010).

Humphries, B. (2004) 'An Unacceptable Role for Social Work: Implementing Immigration Policy', *British Journal of Social Work*, 34: 93–107.

Hunter, J.D. (2000) *The Death of Character: Moral Education in an Age without Good or Evil*, New York: Basic Books.

Illich, I. (1976) *Limits to Medicine: The Expropriation of Health*, Harmondsworth: Penguin.

Illouz, E. (2008) *Saving the Modern Soul: Therapy, Emotions and the Culture of Self-Help*, Berkeley, CA: University of California Press.

Independent Safeguarding Authority (ISA) (2008) 'ISA Scheme Consultation Document: Formal Government Response', 30 May. Available at www.fairplayforchildren.org/pdf/1218024387.pdf (accessed 23 July 2011).

Irvine, E. (1978) 'Psychiatric Social Work: Training for Psychiatric Social Work', in Younghusband, E. (ed.) *Social Work in Britain 1950–1975: A Follow-up Study*, London: Allen & Unwin.

Jacoby, R. (1999) *The End of Utopia: Culture and Politics in an Age of Apathy*, New York: Basic Books.

James, O. (1997) *Britain on the Couch*, London: Century.

Jordan, B. and Parton, N. (1983) *The Political Dimensions of Social Work*, Oxford: Blackwell.

Kirk, S.A. and Kutchins, H. (1997) *Making Us Crazy, DSM: The Psychiatric Bible and the Creation of Mental Disorders*, New York: Aldine de Gruyter.

Klein, N. (2000) *No Logo*, London: HarperCollins.

Knight, K. (2008) 'Posh Protesters: How the Anti-Heathrow Commons Invaders Included a Baronet's Daughter and an MP's Grandson', *Daily Mail*, 29 February. Available at www.dailymail.co.uk/news/article-523220/Posh-protesters-How-anti-Heathrow-Commons-invaders-included-Baronets-granddaughter-MPs-grandson.html (accessed 11 September 2009).

Laing, R.D. (1965) *The Divided Self: An Existential Study in Sanity and Madness*, Harmondsworth: Penguin.

Lane, C. (2007) *Shyness: How Normal Behaviour Became a Sickness*, London: Yale University Press.

Lane, C. (2009) 'Bitterness, Compulsive Shopping and Internet Addiction: The Diagnostic Madness of DSM-V', *Slate*. Available at www.slate.com/id/2223479/ (accessed 4 April 2010).

Langan, M. (2002) 'The Legacy of Radical Social Work', in Adams, R., Dominelli, L. and Payne, M. (eds) *Social Work: Themes, Issues and Critical Debates*, Basingstoke: Palgrave.

Lasch, C. (1979) *The Culture of Narcissism: American Life in an Age of Diminishing Expectations*, New York: Norton.

Lasch, C. (1984) *The Minimal Self: Psychic Survival in Troubled Times*, New York: Norton.

Lasch, C. (1991) 'Afterword', in *The Culture of Narcissism: American Life in an Age of Diminishing Expectations*, new edn, New York: Norton.

Law Commission (1995) *Report on Mental Incapacity*, Report 231, London: The Stationery Office.

Layard, R. (2003) 'Happiness: Has Social Science a Clue?', Lionel Robbins Memorial Lecture, London School of Economics, London.

Layard, R., Seldon, A. and Mulgan, G. (2010) 'Why a Movement for Happiness', *Movement for Happiness*, www.movementforhappiness.org/movement-manifesto/ (accessed 22 November 2010).

Le Bon, G. (1912) *The Psychology of Peoples*, New York: G.E. Stechert.

Lee, E. (2001) 'The Invention of PTSD', *spiked*. Available at www.spiked-online.com/Printable/0000000054B0.htm (accessed 4 October 2010).

Linden, M. (2003) 'Posttraumatic Embitterment Disorder', *Psychotherapy and Psychosomatics*, 72(4): 195–202.

Low, V. (2010) 'Lord Layard's Movement for Happiness Seeks a Director with Vision', *The Times*, 29 March. Available at http://timesonline.co.uk/tol/news/uk/article7079609.ece (accessed 22 November 2010).

Lyotard, J.F. (1989) *The Postmodern Condition: A Report on Knowledge*, Manchester: Manchester University Press.

McAdam, D. (1982) *Political Process and the Development of Black Insurgency 1930–1970*, Chicago, IL: University of Chicago Press.

McCarthy, J.D. and Zald, M.N. (1977) 'Resource Mobilization and Social Movements: A Partial Theory', *American Journal of Sociology*, 82(6): 1212–1241.

McLaughlin, K. (2005) 'One-in-10 Kids are Mentally Ill? That's Madness', *spiked*. Available at www.spiked-online.com/index.php/site/article/445/ (accessed 23 July 2011).

McLaughlin, K. (2008) *Social Work, Politics and Society: From Radicalism to Orthodoxy*, Bristol: Policy Press.

McLaughlin, K. (2010) 'Control and Social Work: A Reflection on Some Twenty-First Century Developments', *Practice*, 22(3): 143–154.

McLaughlin, K. and Appleton, J. (2010) 'Carers or Suspects? CRB Checks and the Regulation of the Caring Professions', *Manifesto Club*. Available at www.manifestoclub.com/files/CarersOrSuspectsReportScreen.pdf (accessed 7 December 2010).

McLaughlin, T. (2002) 'The Trieste Experiment Revisited', *Asylum: The Magazine for Democratic Psychiatry*, 13(2): 3.

McNay, L. (2008) *Against Recognition*, Cambridge: Polity.

Macpherson, W. (1999) *The Stephen Lawrence Inquiry: Report of an Inquiry by Sir William Macpherson of Cluny*, London: HMSO.

Mad Pride (2010) Mad Pride website. Available at www.madpride.org.uk/index.php (accessed 14 September 2010).

Marin, M. (1996) 'Claims that Could Damage a Nation's Health', *Daily Telegraph*, 5 December.

Marx, K. (1978 [1852]) 'The Eighteenth Brumaire of Louis Bonaparte', in Tucker, R.C. (ed.) *The Marx-Engels Reader*, 2nd edn, London: Norton.

Masson, J. (1993) *Against Therapy*, London: HarperCollins.

Melucci, A. (1988) 'Social Movements and the Democratization of Everyday Life', in Keane, J. (ed.) *Civil Society and the State: New European Perspectives*, London: Verso.

Melucci, A. (1995) 'The Process of Collective Identity', in Johnston, H. and Klandermans, B. (eds) *Social Movements and Culture*, London: UCL Press.

Mendel, M.P. (1995) *The Male Survivor: The Impact of Sexual Abuse*, London: Sage.

Mental Health Foundation (MHF) (1999) *The Big Picture*, London: Mental Health Foundation.

Mental Health Foundation (MHF) (2010) 'Fears Over Use of Community Treatment Orders for Mentally Ill'. Available at www.mentalhealth.org.uk/information/news/?EntryId17=81758 (accessed 15 November 2010).

Monbiot, G. (2006) *Heat*, London: Allen Lane.

Monbiot, G. (2008) 'Climate Change is Not Anarchy's Football'. Available at www.guardian.co.uk/commentisfree/2008/aug/22/climatechange.kingsnorth climatecamp (accessed 11 June 2010).

Morris, A. (2004) 'Reflections on Social Movement Theory', in Goodwin, J. and Jasper, J.M. (eds) *Rethinking Social Movements: Structure, Meaning and Emotion*, Oxford: Rowman & Littlefield.

Mullan, B. (1995) *Mad to be Normal: Conversations with R.D. Laing*, London: Free Association Books.

Naess, J. (2010) 'A Question of Trust', *Society Guardian*, 10 November.

National Health Service (NHS) (2010) *NHS Information Centre Statistics*. Available at www.ic.nhs.uk/statistics-and-data-collections/social-care/older-people (accessed 15 November 2010).

Newton, T. (1995) *Managing Stress: Emotion and Power at Work*, London: Sage.

Nolan, J.L. (1998) *The Therapeutic State: Justifying Government at Century's End*, New York: New York University Press.

Novick, P. (1999) *The Holocaust in American Life*, Boston, MA: Houghton Mifflin.

Offe, C. (1987) 'Challenging the Boundaries of Institutional Politics', in Maier, C. (ed.) *Changing the Boundaries of the Political*, Cambridge: Cambridge University Press.

O'Keeffe, M., Hills, A., Doyle, M., McCreadie, C., Scholes, S., Constantine, R., Tinker, A., Manthorpe, J., Biggs, S. and Erens, B. (2007) *UK Study of Abuse and Neglect of Older People: Prevalence Survey Report*, London: Department of Health. Available at http://assets.comicrelief.com/cr09/docs/elderabuseprev.pdf (accessed 23 July 2011).

146   *References*

Oliver, M. (1996) *Understanding Disability: From Theory to Practice*, Basingstoke: Palgrave.

Parker, I. (1989) 'Discourse and Power', in Shotter, J. and Gergen, K.J. (eds) *Texts of Identity*, London: Sage.

Parker, I. (2001) 'Psychology, Politics, Resistance: Asylum in the 21st Century', *Asylum: The Magazine for Democratic Psychiatry*, 13(1): 14–15.

Parker, I. (2007) *Revolution in Psychology: Alienation to Emancipation*, London: Pluto.

Parker, I., Georgaca, E., Harper, D., McLaughlin, T. and Stowell, M.S. (1995) *Deconstructing Psychopathology*, London: Sage.

Parsons, T. (1978) *Action Theory and the Human Condition*, New York: Free Press.

Patmore, A. (2006) *The Truth about Stress*, London: Atlantic Books.

Phillips, A. (2008) 'From Inequality to Difference: A Severe Case of Displacement', in Fraser, N., *Adding Insult to Injury: Nancy Fraser Debates her Critics* (edited by K. Olsen), London: Verso.

Pilgrim, D. and Rogers, A. (1999) *A Sociology of Mental Health and Illness*, 2nd edn, Buckingham: Open University Press.

Pringle, M. and Laverty, J. (1993) 'A Counsellor in Every Practice?', *British Medical Journal*, 306(6869): 2–3.

Pupavac, V. (2001) 'Therapeutic Governance: Psychosocial Intervention and Trauma Risk Management', *Disasters*, 25(4): 358–372.

Rieff, P. (1966) *The Triumph of the Therapeutic: Uses of Faith after Freud*, New York: Harper.

Roberts, J. (2007) 'Ex-Gay Survivors Speak Out', *Pink News*, 29 June. Available at www.pinknews.co.uk/news/articles/2005-4795.html (accessed 7 April 2008).

Rorty, R. (2008) 'Is "Cultural Recognition" a Useful Notion for Leftist Politics?', in Fraser, N., *Adding Insult to Injury: Nancy Fraser Debates her Critics* (edited by K. Olsen), London: Verso.

Sanders, T. (2009) 'Kerbcrawler Rehabilitation Programmes: Curing the "Deviant Male" and Reinforcing the "Respectable" Moral Order', *Critical Social Policy*, 29: 77–99.

Sawicki, J. (1991) *Disciplining Foucault: Feminism, Power and the Body*, London: Routledge.

Sayce, L. (2000) *From Psychiatric Patient to Citizen*, Basingstoke: Palgrave.

Scott, W. (1990) 'PTSD in DSM-III: A Case in the Politics of Diagnosis and Disease', *Social Problems*, 37(3): 294–310.

Shakespeare, T. (1993) 'Disabled People's Self-Organization: A New Social Movement?', *Disability, Handicap and Society*, 8(3): 249–264.

Short, C. (2009) 'The Forces Shaping Radical Politics Today', in Pugh, J. (ed.) *What is Radical Politics Today?*, Basingstoke: Palgrave Macmillan.

Showalter, E. (1987) *The Female Malady*, London: Virago.

Showalter, E. (1997) *Hystories: Hysterical Epidemics and Modern Culture*, New York: Columbia University Press.

Simon, B. (2004) *Identity in Modern Society: A Social and Psychological Perspective*, Oxford: Blackwell.

Smail, D. (1996) *How to Survive without Psychotherapy*, London: Constable.

Snow, D.A. (1992) 'Master Frames and Cycles of Protest', in Morris, A.D. and McClurg Mueller, C. (eds) *Frontiers in Social Movement Theory*, New Haven, CT: Yale University Press.

Snow, D.A., Soule, S.A. and Hanspeter, K. (eds) (2007a) *The Blackwell Companion to Social Movements*, Oxford: Blackwell.

Snow, D.A., Soule, S.A. and Hanspeter, K. (2007b) 'Mapping the Terrain', in Snow, D.A., Soule, S.A. and Hanspeter, K. (eds) *The Blackwell Companion to Social Movements*, Oxford: Blackwell.

Snow, R. (2002) *Stronger Than Ever: The Report of the First National Conference of Survivor Workers UK*, Stockport: Asylum.

Sontag, S. (1989) *Illness as Metaphor and AIDS and its Metaphors*, New York: Doubleday.

Spandler, H. (2006) *Asylum to Action: Paddington Day Hospital, Therapeutic Communities and Beyond*, London: Jessica Kingsley.

Spandler, H. and Batsleer, J. (2000) 'Sparring Partners', in Batsleer, J. and Humphries, B. (eds) *Welfare, Exclusion and Political Agency*, London: Routledge.

Speed, E. (2006) 'Patients, Consumers and Survivors: A Case Study of Mental Health Service User Discourses', *Social Science and Medicine*, 62: 28–38.

Spicker, P. (2006) *Liberty, Equality, Fraternity*, Bristol: Policy Press.

Stein, A. (2007) 'Trauma Stories, Identity Work, and the Politics of Recognition', in Gregson, J.M. and Wolf, D.L. (eds) *Sociology Confronts the Holocaust: Memories and Identities in Jewish Diasporas*, Durham, NC: Duke University Press.

Stein, A. (2009) 'Feminism, Therapeutic Culture and the Holocaust in the United States: The Second Generation Phenomenon', *Jewish Social Studies: History, Culture, Society*, n.s. 16(1): 27–53.

Stewart, J. (2009) 'The Scientific Claims of British Child Guidance, 1918–45', *British Journal for the History of Science*, 42: 407–432.

Stratton, A. (2009) 'Jobless to be Offered "Talking Treatment" to Help Put Britain Back to Work', *Guardian*, 4 December. Available at www.guardian.co.uk/society/2009/dec/04/jobless-therapy-talking-cbt-unemployment (accessed 13 October 2010).

Stratton, A. (2010) 'David Cameron Aims to Make Happiness the New GDP', *Guardian*, 14 November. Available at www.guardian.co.uk/politics/2010/nov/14/david-cameron-wellbeing-inquiry/print (accessed 22 November 2010).

Summerfield, D. (1996) *The Impact of War and Atrocity on Civilian Populations: Basic Principles for NGO Interventions and a Critique of Psychosocial Trauma Project*s, London: Overseas Development Institute.

Swingewood, A. (2000) *A Short History of Sociological Thought*, 3rd edn, Basingstoke: Palgrave.

Szasz, T.S. (1961) *The Myth of Mental Illness: Foundations of a Theory of Personal Conduct*, New York: Dell.

Szasz, T.S. (1976) 'Anti-Psychiatry: The Paradigm of the Plundered Mind', *New Review*, 3: 3–14.

Szasz, T.S. (1991) *Ideology and Insanity: Essays on the Psychiatric Dehumanization of Man*, Syracuse, NY: Syracuse University Press.

Szasz, T.S. (2010) 'The Role of Psychiatry in the Therapeutic State', *Asylum: The Magazine for Democratic Psychiatry*, 17(3): 3–4.

Tarrow, S. (1994) *Power in Movement: Social Movements, Collective Action and Politics*, Cambridge: Cambridge University Press.

Tarrow, S. (1998) *Power in Movement: Social Movements, Collective Action and Politics*, 2nd edn, Cambridge: Cambridge University Press.

Taylor, C. (1994) 'The Politics of Recognition', in Guttman, A. (ed.) *Multiculturalism: Examining the Politics of Recognition*, Princeton, NJ: Princeton University Press.

Thomas. P. (1997) *The Dialectics of Schizophrenia*, London: Free Association Books.

Thompson, A. (1999) 'No Fear: Danger Zone', *Community Care*, 22–28 July: 24–25.

Tilly, C. (1995) 'Contentious Repertoires in Great Britain, 1758–1834', in Traugott, M. (ed.) *Repertoires and Cycles of Contention*, Durham, NC: Duke University Press.

Tomes, N. (2006) 'The Patient as a Policy Factor: A Historical Case Study of the Consumer/Survivor Movement in Mental Health', *Regulation and Policy*, May–June: 720–729.

Trades Union Congress (TUC) (2008) *Hard Work, Hidden Lives: The Full Report of the Commission on Vulnerable Employment*, London: College Hill Press. Available at www.vulnerableworkers.org.uk/files/CoVE_full_report.pdf (accessed 1 June 2010).

United Nations Development Programme (UNDP) (1999) *Human Development Report 1999*, New York: UNDP.

University of the West of England (UWE) (2009) 'Climate Change Denial Conference Hosted at UWE'. Available at http://info.uwe.ac.uk/news/UWENews/article.asp?item=1438 (accessed 20 January 2010).

Upham, M. (ed.) (1996) *Trade Unions of the World*, 4th edn, London: Cartermill.

Wainwright, D. and Calnan, M. (2002) *Work Stress: The Making of a Modern Epidemic*, Buckingham: Open University Press.

Walia, S. (2004) '"Spectres of Derrida": Obituary of Jacques Derrida', *Frontline*, 21(23). Available at www.hinduonnet.com/fline/fl2123/stories/20041119007712800.htm (accessed 29 April 2010).

Weaver, H.N. and Burns, B. (2001) '"I Shout with Fear at Night": Understanding the Traumatic Experiences of Refugees and Asylum Seekers', *Journal of Social Work*, 1: 147–164.

Wetherell, M. and Potter, J. (1992) *Mapping the Language of Racism: Discourse and the Legitimation of Exploitation*, Hemel Hempstead: Harvester Wheatsheaf.

Wilkomirski, B. (1996) *Fragments: Memories of a Wartime Childhood*, trans. Janeway, C.B., New York: Schocken.

Williams, F. (1999) 'Good-Enough Principles for Welfare', *Journal of Social Policy*, 28(4): 667–687.

Wilson, J. (1973) *Introduction to Social Movements*, New York: Basic Books.

Wolf, D.L. (2007) 'Holocaust Testimony: Producing Post-Memories, Producing Identities', in Gregson, J.M and Wolf, D.L. (eds) *Sociology Confronts the Holocaust: Memories and Identities in Jewish Diasporas*, Durham, NC: Duke University Press.

Wolf, S. (1994) 'Comment', in Gutmann, A. (ed.) *Multiculturalism: Examining the Politics of Recognition*, Oxford: Oxford University Press.

World Health Organization (WHO) (1965) *International Statistical Classification of Diseases and Related Health Problems* (ICD-8). Geneva: WHO.

Ziegenmeyer, N. (1992) *Taking Back My Life*, New York: Simon & Schuster.

Index

McLaughlin, K. and Appleton, J. 120
McNay, L. 41, 46, 47–8
Mad Pride 3, 15, 87, 92, 93, 108
Marx, K. 12
Marxist theory 41, 43
the masses *see* working class
Masson, J. 88
meaning 29–30
medical discourse 88–9
medical insurance 109–10
Melucci, A. 134
memory: collective 69; post-memory 56; recovered/false 65
Mental Health Act 73n3, 83, 84–5, 98
Mental Health Foundation 101
mental illness 75–6, 77, 101–2 *see also* anti-psychiatry; psychiatric survival; class and mental distress 91; and compensation claims 109–10; pathologizing of dissent 102; recognizing madness 88–90; and terminology 84–8; and therapeutic identity *see* therapeutic identity; and the transformation of the sick role 108–10
Mental Patients Union (MPU) 79, 87; 'Fish Manifesto' 91
middle class 23, 24, 26
Mind 102
MINDLINK 80
miners' strike 24, 34, 115–16
misrecognition 37, 38, 39, 41, 42, 45–7, 89, 96, 129
Monbiot, G. 25
Morris, A. 15
movement culture 14–15
Movement for Happiness 130–4, 135n3
MPU *see* Mental Patients Union
Mulgan, Geoff 131, 133

Naess, J. 117
National Council for Mental Hygiene 76
national identity 32
Nazi Holocaust *see* Holocaust
neglect 125
neo-liberalism 134
New Labour 30, 114–15, 130, 131

new social movements (NSMs) 19–24, 40, 44, 133–5; Happiness Movement 130–4; user/survivor movement 74, 79–84, 86–7, 90, 92
Newton, T. 117
NIMBY (not in my back yard) groups 10
No Secrets 119
Nolan, J. L. 108
non-conformity 19–20 *see also* social movements
normalcy 62
Northern Ireland 61
Novick, P. 69
NSMs *see* new social movements

objectification 43, 77, 84, 95
Offe, C. 24, 134
O'Keeffe, M. et al. 125
Oliver, Jamie 133–4
Oliver, M. 23
One Flew Over the Cuckoo's Nest 78
Optimum Population Trust 25, 26

Paddington Day Hospital 79
Parker, I. et al. 83–4
Parks, Rosa 15
Parsons, T. 108
Patmore, A. 114, 115
performativity, theory of 98, 99
pharmaceutical industry 103–4, 111
Phillips, A. 44
Pol Pot 31
police checks 122–4, 125–6
politics *see also* Conservative Party; New Labour: and austerity 25; collapse of left/right ideologies 24, 25, 28, 115; decline of working class political organization 22–7, 28; depoliticization of state actions 27, 121; downgrading of Political issues 121; ethnic 56; evacuation of the masses/working class from 24, 28; of fear 8, 112–13, 122; gay 10; green 24; and the Happiness Movement 130–4; identity *see* identity politics; and the imposition of vulnerable identity 112–13, 114–17, 121, 127; interest in identity 2–3; and justice *see* social

verbal abuse 52
Viagra 103
victimization/victimhood 33, 51, 55,
59, 60, 61, 69; breaking the silence
56, 64–8, 72; Holocaust
victimhood 55–8; privileging of
victim testimony 68–9, 70; rape
victims/survivors 62, 64, 66;
refusal to embrace victim identity
69
Vine, Jeremy 105
vulnerability 7–8, 112–27; and
abuse of adults 124–6; and
autonomy 27; and disdain 27;
fundamental 38; imposition of a
vulnerable identity 112–27; and
the Independent Safeguarding
Authority 27, 120, 123; legal
construction of the vulnerable
adult 118–21; official
classification of the vulnerable
118; and protection 27, 113–14,
116, 121–4; stress and the role of
trade unions 114–18

Wainwright, D. and Calnan, M.
99–100, 115–16
Walia, S. 99

welfare: active welfare subjects 22–3;
benefit cuts 130; campaign to
protect benefits 93; general well-
being and the Happiness
Movement 130–4; systems 20–1
Wetherell, M. and Potter, J. 99
Wilkomirski, B. 58
Williams, F. 22–3
Wilson, J. 10
women's exploitation 43
women's groups 36
women's rights 26
Woolf, Virginia 26
work stress 105, 114, 115–16, 116
working class 22, 23, 24, 26, 33, 34–5,
41, 43, 91–2, 133; contempt for the
masses 26–7, 28, 133–4; and the
defeat of the miners' strike 115–16;
moving against the masses 23–7;
politics 21, 22–7, 28, 93, 115–16;
withdrawal from politics 24, 28,
115–16
workplace bullying 116

Zerubavel, E. 66
Zito, Jayne 70
Zito Trust 70, 73n3
Zurn, C. 41